AF545112

Clinical Use of the Palmaz-Schatz Intracoronary Stent

Edited by

Howard C. Herrmann, MD
Director, Interventional Cardiology
Hospital of the University of Pennsylvania
Associate Professor of Medicine
University of Pennsylvania School of Medicine
Philadelphia, Pennsylvania

and

John W. Hirshfeld, Jr., MD
Director, Cardiac Catheterization Laboratory
Hospital of the University of Pennsylvania
Professor of Medicine
University of Pennsylvania School of Medicine
Philadelphia, Pennsylvania

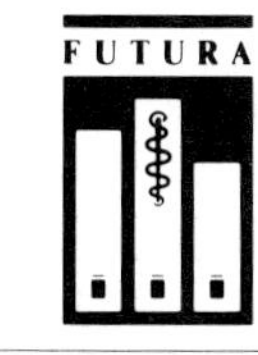

Futura Publishing Company, Inc.
Mount Kisco, NY

Library of Congress Cataloging-in-Publication Data

Clinical use of the Palmaz-Schatz intracoronary
stent/ edited by Howard C. Herrmann and John W. Hirshfeld, Jr.
p. cm.
Includes bibliographical references and index.
ISBN 0-87993-565-0
1. Stents (Surgery) 2. Transluminal angioplasty. 3. Coronary
arteries—Diseases—Treatment. I. Herrmann, Howard C.
II. Hirshfeld, John W.
[DNLM: 1. Angioplasty, Transluminal, Percutaneous Coronary.
2. Coronary Disease—therapy. 3. Stents. WG 300 C6415 1993]
RD598.35.S73C45 1993
617.4′12059—dc20
DNLM/DLC
for Library of Congress 93-11237
CIP

Published by
Futura Publishing Company, Inc.
2 Bedford Ridge Road
P.O. Box 330
Mount Kisco, New York 10549

L.C. No.: 93-11237
ISBN No.: 0-87993-565-0

Every effort has been made to ensure that the information in this book is as up to date and accurate as possible at the time of publication. However, due to the constant developments in medicine, neither the author, nor the editor, nor the publisher can accept any legal or any other responsibility for any errors or omissions that may occur.

Printed in the United States of America on acid-free paper.

To our wives, Deborah and Barbara
for their support and encouragement

Contributors

Donald S. Baim, M.D.
Director, Invasive Cardiology, Beth Israel Hospital, Associate Professor of Medicine, Harvard Medical School, Boston, Massachusetts

Elliot S. Barnathan, M.D.
Director, Vascular Biology Program, Hospital of the University of Pennsylvania, Assistant Professor of Medicine, University of Pennsylvania School of Medicine, Philadelphia, Pennsylvania

Robert F. Bonner, Ph.D.
Washington Hospital Center, Washington, DC

Joseph P. Carrozza, Jr., M.D.
Director, Interventional Animal Research, Beth Israel Hospital, Instructor in Medicine, Harvard Medical School, Boston, Massachusetts

Stephen A. Downing, M.D.
Chief Resident, General Surgery, Hospital of the University of Pennsylvania, University of Pennsylvania School of Medicine, Philadelphia, Pennsylvania

Stephen G. Ellis, M.D.
Director, Sones Cardiac Catheterization Laboratory, Cleveland Clinic Foundation, Cleveland, Ohio

David L. Fischman, M.D.
Assistant Professor of Medicine, Thomas Jefferson University Hospital, Jefferson Medical College, Philadelphia, Pennsylvania

Sheldon Goldberg, M.D.
Director, Division of Cardiology, Thomas Jefferson University Hospital, Professor of Medicine, Jefferson Medical College, Philadelphia, Pennsylvania

Michael A. Golden, M.D.
Assistant Professor of Surgery, Hospital of the University of Pennsylvania, University of Pennsylvania School of Medicine, Philadelphia, Pennsylvania

Howard C. Herrmann, M.D.
Director, Interventional Cardiology, Hospital of the University of Pennsylvania, Associate Professor of Medicine, University of Pennsylvania School of Medicine, Philadelphia, Pennsylvania

John W. Hirshfeld, Jr., M.D.
Director, Cardiac Catheterization Laboratory, Hospital of the University of Pennsylvania, Professor of Medicine, University of Pennsylvania School of Medicine, Philadelphia, Pennsylvania

Gad Keren, M.D.
Washington Hospital Center, Washington, D.C.

Martin B. Leon, M.D.
Director, Investigational Angioplasty Program, Washington Hospital Center, Washington, D.C.

Gary S. Mintz, M.D.
Washington Hospital Center, Washington, D.C.

Julio C. Palmaz, M.D.
Chief, Cardiovascular and Special Interventions, Professor of Radiology, University of Texas Health Science Center, San Antonio, Texas

Augusto D. Pichard, M.D.
Director, Cardiac Catheterization Laboratory, Washington Hospital Center, Washington, D.C.

Jeffrey J. Popma, M.D.
Washington Hospital Center, Washington, D.C.

Michael P. Savage, M.D.
Director, Cardiac Catheterization Laboratory, Thomas Jefferson University Hospital, Assistant Professor of Medicine, Jefferson Medical College, Philadelphia, Pennsylvania

Richard A. Schatz, M.D.
Research Director, Cardiovascular Interventions, Scripps Clinic and Research Foundation, La Jolla, California

Shing-Chiu Wong, M.D.
Washington Hospital Center, Washington, D.C.

Andrew Zalewski, M.D.
Director, Interventional Cardiology Research, Thomas Jefferson University Hospital, Associate Professor of Medicine, Jefferson Medical College, Philadelphia, Pennsylvania

Foreword

The field of interventional cardiology has developed rapidly over the past decade. The early investigators in this field did not predict either the rapid growth of this procedure or the emergence and wide use of new devices with the potential to enhance conventional percutaneous transluminal coronary angioplasty.

The introduction of new techniques and devices to relieve coronary stenoses has presented the interventional cardiologist with a flood of new information which must be applied to clinical practice. This requires the interventionalist to be highly adaptable, constantly learning, and available for re-training. This sort of information is generally not assembled in an organized fashion in the various periodicals related to this field.

It was the need for a comprehensive organized source of information about the Palmaz-Schatz balloon-expandable intracoronary stent that prompted us to undertake the editing of this monograph. In particular, our purpose was to provide a handbook for interventional cardiologists who plan to use the Palmaz-Schatz intracoronary stent; essentially, a one-stop source of information on the design, indications, complications, acute and long-term results, and technical aspects of insertion of this new device. We hope that this book will be used in conjunction with observational live-demonstration courses and other "hands-on" experiences prior to a cardiologist's first attempt at stent implantation.

We are grateful to all of the Palmaz-Schatz investigators who helped gather the data described in the book, many of whom also contributed as authors. We are also indebted to Steven Korn, Zita Jackson, and Lucille O'Connor for their assistance in publishing, typing, and editing this work. Finally, we hope that this book will be of sufficient use to practicing interventional cardiologists, and that future editions can be published and updated as new information on this emerging technology becomes available.

Howard C. Herrmann, M.D.
John W. Hirshfeld, Jr., M.D.
Philadelphia, Pennsylvania

Table of Contents

V Future Directions and Conclusions

I

Background

CHAPTER 1

Developmental Background and Design of the Palmaz-Schatz Coronary Stents

Shing-Chiu Wong
Richard A. Schatz

In 1964 Dotter introduced the technique of peripheral angioplasty by using successively larger catheters to enlarge obstructive vascular lesions.[1] In the same landmark article, he also proposed the concept of using endovascular prostheses postangioplasty as a conduit to maintain an adequate channel until the natural reendothelialization process took place. In retrospect, both ideas reflected Dotter's tremendous insight into the pathophysiology of obstructive vascular disease and paved the way for the development of modern interventional cardiology. He subsequently reported his experience on the use of stainless steel and nitinol coils in peripheral arteries of dogs.[2,3]

Another milestone of modern interventional cardiology was established in 1977 when Gruentzig reported on his innovative use of balloon catheters for the treatment of obstructive coronary lesions.[4] In the subsequent 15 years, there has been a tremendous growth in the volume of angioplasty with accummulation of operator experience, and refinement of balloon, guidewire, and guiding catheter designs.[5,6] This has resulted in a definite improvement in the rate of initial angioplasty success.[7] On the other hand, despite intense effort and a multitude of pharmacologic trials in the last decade, solutions to prevent acute closure and chronic restenosis remain elusive.

In addition to the morbidity and mortality associated with acute vascular occlusion and restenosis, the economic and psychological toll experienced by both physicians and patients has provided the impetus for research and development of new devices to treat these two persistent problems. Thus, the two goals for the development of stent technology are: to prevent and treat acute closure, and to reduce the incidence of chronic restenosis.

In this chapter, we will outline the history of stent technology, possible

From: Herrmann HC, Hirshfeld JW, eds. *Clinical Use of the Palmaz-Schatz Intracoronary Stent.* Futura Publishing Company, Inc., Mount Kisco, NY, © 1993.

mechanisms to explain why stents may help treat acute closure and prevent chronic restenosis, a description of the evolution of designs that led to the current generation of the Johnson & Johnson Palmaz-Schatz stent (Johnson & Johnson Interventional Systems, Warren, NJ), the preclinical data that preceded clinical trials of the Palmaz-Schatz stent, as well as limitations and future developments in stent technology.

History of Stent Development

The term "stent" is derived from a nineteenth-century British dentist, Charles R. Stent, who invented dental impression material that was later used to support healing skin grafts. Subsequently, any device that is used to maintain a body cavity during skin grafting is referred to as a stent. Dotter first introduced the concept of an endovascular "splint" in 1964.[1] He reported his initial experience with a spring coil in an animal model in 1969[2,3] and, later, experience with a nitinol endovascular prosthesis in 1983.[3,8] Other investigators who helped to lay the groundwork for current stents included Maas who designed a spiral double-helix stainless-steel spring,[9] and Wright who described a zig-zag pattern spring stent.[10]

Palmaz was the first to design a stent based on balloon expansion for deployment.[11] With the tremendous growth of balloon- angioplasty techniques and equipment in the past decade, the marriage of stent and balloon catheter technologies seemed only natural. A logical offspring of the initial successful preclinical[12] and subsequent clinical experience[13] in the peripheral vasculature is its application to the coronary vasculature.

Possible Mechanisms to Prevent Acute Closure and Chronic Restenosis

The incidence of acute closure following balloon angioplasty is about 7%.[14] It is associated with a 4.9% in-hospital mortality and 4.1% additional out of hospital mortality, despite emergency bypass surgery.[14] It is believed that acute closure results largely from plaque disruption and dissection, with subsequent spasm and thrombosis. Therefore, stents provide a logical solution for scaffolding and sealing the disrupted intimal/medial flap. All the stents that are currently available have been successfully deployed for this purpose, with good results.[15,16] The use of stents for acute occlusion after angioplasty is discussed in Chapter 6.

Restenosis after successful angioplasty occurs in 30% to 40% of patients with native coronary lesions,[17–19] and in up to 70% of patients with saphenous vein grafts.[20,21] Early restenosis during the first few days postangioplasty may occur in as many as 11% of lesions due to elastic recoil, vasospasm, platelet-fibrin thrombi deposition, or a combination of these factors.[22–24] Rensing et al used a quantitative videodensitometric technique to analyze the difference between balloon cross-sectional area and minimal luminal area after percutaneous transluminal coronary angioplasty (PTCA) in 136 patients with 151 lesions. They reported a 50% reduction in the theoretically achievable cross-sectional area immediately postangioplasty, which was attributed to elastic recoil.[25]

By providing mechanical support after dilatation, stents can significantly reduce or eliminate the amount of vascular recoil postdilatation.[26,27] The relatively smooth endoluminal surface after stent placement may reduce turbulence and improve regional flow characteristics. Elimination of vessel areas with turbulent flow can reduce low-arterial wall shear stress, which may contribute to intimal thickening.[28,29]

Finally, by sealing the exposed subintimal spaces, stents may minimize local thrombosis which contributes to the organization and subsequent conversion of platelet-fibrin complexes into the restenosis plaque. It is possible that a reduction in the amount of subintimal exposure could also reduce the activation of smooth muscle cells and the release of growth factors.[15]

Desirable Characteristics of a Stent

Table 1 summarizes the desirable characteristics of an ideal stent. In order to reach the target lesion, a stent must be flexible enough to negotiate through the bends and curves of guiding catheters and coronary vessels. On the other hand, a stent must also be strong enough to withstand circumferential collapse despite potentially millions of cycles of cardiac contractions after deployment. These properties are determined by the elastic limit and modulus of the metal, as well as the stent configuration,[30] and are discussed in more detail in Chapter 12.

The ideal metallic stent needs to be minimally thrombogenic. Electronega-

Table 1.
Desirable Characteristics of an "Ideal" Stent

1. Low profile
2. Longitudinally flexible
3. Radially noncompliant
4. Thromboresistant
5. Corrosion-resistant
6. Mechanically durable
7. Good flouroscopic visibility
8. High-expansion ratio
9. Reliably expandable
10. Complete wall contact

tive metals are relatively thromboresistant, but are very susceptible to corrosion. Unfortunately, most metals, including stainless steel, are electropositive and therefore thrombogenic. Furthermore, thrombogenicity may also be related to the metal thickness and porosity.[31] Thus, a metal stent should have minimal surface area, be low profile, corrosion-resistant, and durable.[32]

Current stainless-steel stents have poor visibility under fluoroscopy because of the small mass. This limitation can compromise the precision of stent placement and its recovery if dislodgement during deployment occurs. Tantalum is more radiopaque and has elastic properties that make it suitable for use in balloon-expandable stents. However, the advantages of tantalum may be offset by its mechanical fragility and propensity for stress fracture.

Optimal matching between the stent and vessel size is important for securing the stent in place once it is deployed. Underexpansion may allow migration and embolization, whereas overstretching may cause intimal or medial trauma.[33] Of the three stent designs that are currently available, balloon-expandable stents appear to have an advantage in precise expansion control by the operator during the procedure.

Finally, an ideal stent should have the largest expansion ratio possible without compromising its structural strength. This will help minimize the profile of the stent-delivery system and allow for precise stent-to-artery matching over a wide range of operating diameters. This assures optimal wall contact which is likely to be important in reducing thrombosis and restenosis.

Stent Designs

There are currently three basic stent designs available for coronary artery implantation:

1. The spring-loaded self-expanding type stent consists of an elastic woven wire-mesh tube that can adapt to variable diameters and still maintain its radial expansion force. It is constrained to a small diameter by a membrane on the end of a delivery catheter. After the stent-delivery catheter reaches its target, the constraining membrane is removed, allowing the stent to expand radially to a predetermined diameter. An example of this type of stent is the Medinvent stent which was developed jointly by the University Hospital at Lausanne and Medinvent Inc. in Switzerland,[34] (Fig. 1, upper panel). The advantages of such a design include its geometric stability and its flexibility.

2. Nitinol stents are representative of the thermal expansion type. Nitinol is able to change its configuration when exposed to heat. Thus, it can be mounted in a coil on a small-diameter catheter for delivery to the site of stenosis. After warming, the metal coil will assume a predetermined shape. Despite its initial report by Dotter and Craggs as early as 1983,[3,8] the complex delivery process and unpredictable rate of expansion have limited the experience with this type of stent.

3. Palmaz and colleagues introduced the third type of balloon-expandable stainless-steel stent design in 1984.[11] The delivery and implantation of this

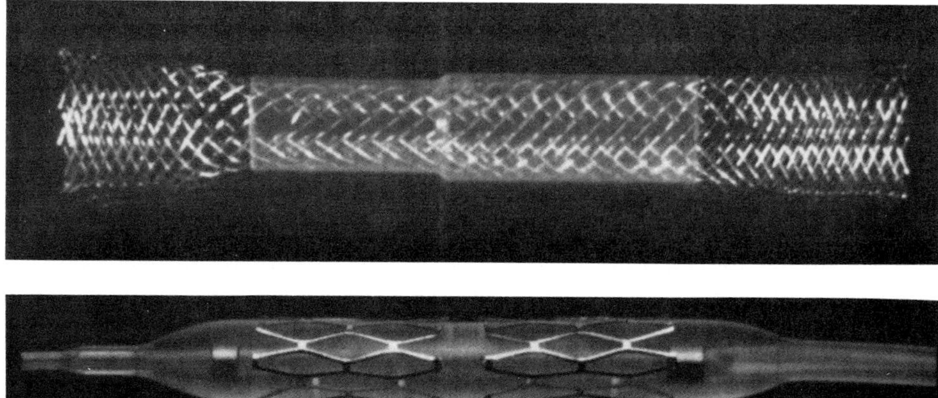

Figure 1: *Medinvent stent (upper panel) and Palmaz-Schatz stent (lower panel).*

stent makes use of the metallic property of plastic deformity whereby it will not change its shape once it is stretched beyond its elastic limit. The advantages of this particular design include its low profile and minimal metal surface area. A balloon catheter-based delivery system enables relatively easy, precise, and reliable deployment. However, the original Palmaz single-tubular inflexible design hindered its deployment in the coronary system. A subsequent modification into two shorter segments joined by an articulated strut has largely overcome this problem (Fig. 1, lower panel).

Composition, Configuration, and Basic Design Characteristics of the Palmaz-Schatz Coronary Stent

The initial Palmaz stent prototype was constructed by using a continuous woven stainless-steel wire of 0.15 mm in diameter to construct 4-, 5-, 6-, and 8-mm grafts, and 0.2-mm wire for the 10-mm stent, with cross-points soldered with silver. The grafts were manually compressed and crimped over a balloon-angioplasty catheter. Multiple animal studies were conducted and showed excellent compatibility and patency results (see below.[35–38])

Later, the continuous woven-wire construct was replaced by a stainless-steel tubular design. The modified Palmaz balloon-expandable stent is a surgical-grade, monoconstructed slotted stainless-steel tube with a 0.08-mm wall thickness. The coronary design is available as a single 15-mm long segment for small arteries which is expandable up to 6 mm in diameter. Devices for other vessels include a 20-mm long articulated stent which is expandable to a 9-mm diameter for use in medium-sized arteries, and a 30-mm long stent for larger arteries which can be expanded to 18 mm.

The walls of the redesigned stent are etched into multiple rows of staggered rectangular slots that assume a diamond shape upon expansion. At typical expanded diameters, the metal occupies only 10% of the total vessel surface area. This version of stent not only minimizes the amount of metal surface without compromising the radial strength of the stent, but it may also allow multiple foci of endothelium to protrude through the interstices to facilitate rapid reendothelialization.[39]

The single segment rigid tubular design was difficult to pass through the bends of guiding catheters and serpiginous coronary arteries. The flexibility of the stent-delivery system improved considerably with the introduction of a central 1-mm articulating bridge between two 7-mm rigid segments. This modified stent design is referred to as the Palmaz-Schatz stent. Improvement in the flexibility with the articulated design overcomes only part of the hurdle of the stent-delivery process. The stent mounted over a balloon catheter is still exposed to the often tortuous arterial segments proximal to the target site, as well as the sometimes dissected or ulcerated lesion within the target site. This can result in suboptimal placement or embolization of the stent during deployment.[40,41] The introduction of a protective sheath mounted over the stent and balloon-catheter system has greatly enhanced the safety of stent delivery.[41] The current system is described in more detail in Chapter 2.

In Vivo Experimental Data on the Palmaz-Schatz Stent

The effects of intra-arterial stenting using a continuous woven stainless-steel wire prototype were first examined in dogs by Palmaz and his colleagues.[35,37] They noted partial thrombosis in several nonheparinized dogs, but no thrombosis was observed in animals receiving systemic heparinization. In these early experiments, the researchers also observed more intimal hyperplasia within stents placed in smaller caliber vessels and in vessels with outflow obstruction. Histopathologic analysis revealed that there was an orderly sequence of events that led to the final endothelization of the implanted stent. Within hours after stent deployment, a concentric layer of red thrombus was deposited over the device, and was replaced with a thin layer of fibrin coating by 1 week (Fig. 2A). Light microscopy revealed early organization of fibrin on the luminal surface of the stent (Fig. 2B), and electron microscopy showed early but incomplete endothelialization by immature endothelial cells with bulging nuclei on the luminal surface of the stent (Fig. 2C).

The fibrin deposit was replaced by a translucent endothelialized neointima by 3 weeks (Fig. 3A), and the media was partially replaced by fibrocollagenous tissue (Fig. 3B). At the same time, the inflammatory response in the adventitia began to subside. By 8 weeks, the neointima showed further organization; the endoluminal surface of the stent was covered by a whitish, opalescent layer, visible by gross inspection with further organization microscopically (Fig. 4).

Finally, by 32 weeks after stent implantation, the neointima became thinner and appeared less cellular, with more intercellular ground substance. Hemosiderin pigments were visible, and the media was thinner, especially at sites

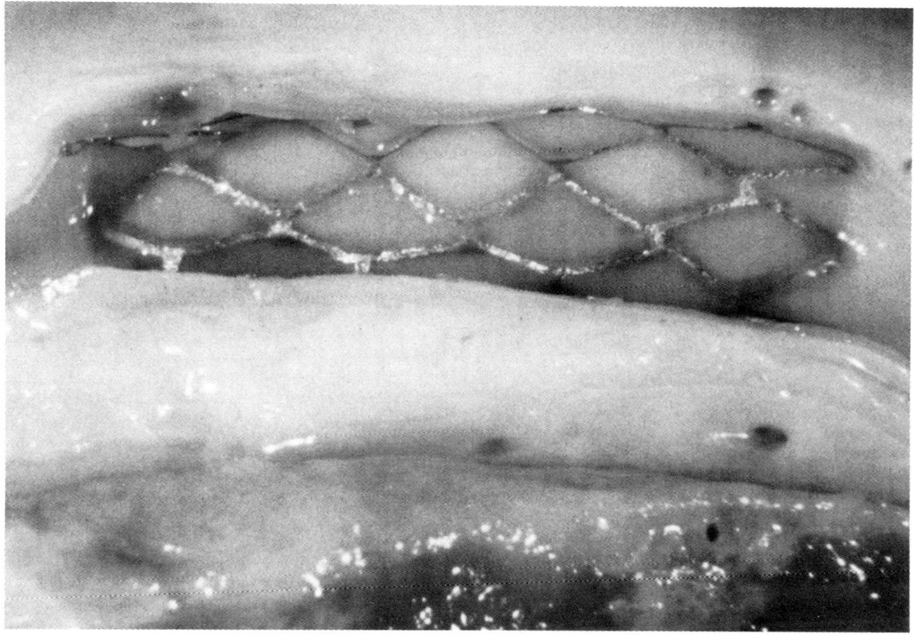

Figure 2A: *In vivo experimental histology after stent implantation. At 1 week, on gross specimen, the stent is easily seen through a thin layer of neointima.*

beneath the stent struts (Figs. 5A, 5B). On scanning electron microscopy, the endothelial cells first arranged in the direction of flow by the third week, but continued to mature and transformed into flat, elongated cells aligned in the direction of the blood flow by 32 weeks (Fig. 5C).

Stent Design Revision

The relatively large profile of the initial stent prototype, especially at the wire intersection points, hampered stent delivery in small vessels. As a result, Palmaz replaced it with a more streamlined slotted-tube design with a lower profile and smoother surface. Subsequent deployment of this stent in multiple animal models including atherosclerotic rabbit aortas and normal and stenotic renal arteries of dogs and pigs was achieved with close to a 100% patency rate.[36,38] A similar sequence of endothelialization was observed by gross inspection, light and electron microscopy, and by factor VII-related antigen assay.[35–38]

To examine the short- and long-term response to the Palmaz vascular stent, Schatz and colleagues stented the coronary arteries of normal dogs. The animals were pretreated with dipyridamole and aspirin 1 day prior to stenting, and with heparin and dextran during the procedure. This anticoagulation pro-

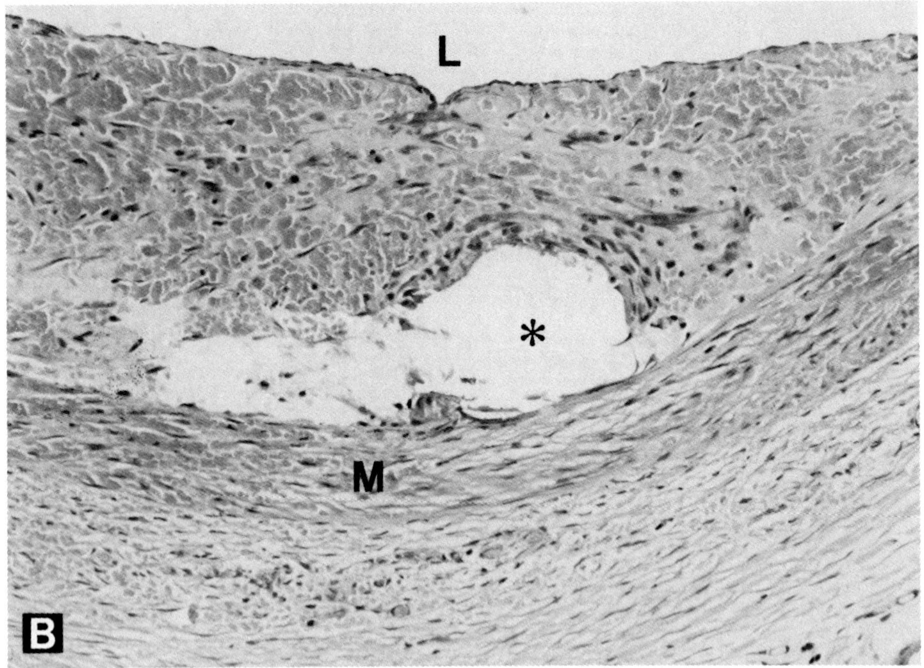

Figure 2B: *In vivo experimental histology after stent implantation. Immature endothelial cells cover thrombus and fibrin deposition on the stent. (* = stent; L = lumen; M = media.)*

tocol was based on a previous set of experiments performed in 64 dogs, testing the antithrombotic efficacy of different medical regimens.[42] Heparin alone was compared with heparin, aspirin, plus dipyridamole, and with heparin, aspirin, dipyridamole, plus dextran. By measuring the amount of radioactive 111-indium-labeled platelet deposit in the stented sites, the researchers noted a maximal decrease in platelets and fibrin deposition when dextran was used in conjunction with heparin, aspirin, and dipyridamole.[42]

Stents were deployed in canine left anterior descending, left main, or circumflex coronary arteries with follow-up angiography obtained at 1, 3, 6, and 12 months. The animals were also sacrificed in groups of three at 1, 3, 8, and 32 weeks for gross-, light-, and electron-microscopic analysis. All dogs survived until sacrifice, and all stent sites were found to be patent without spasm, rupture, or aneurysm formation. Histopathologic analysis and electron microscopy of the stented sites again showed an orderly progression of thrombus deposition, with subsequent reendothelialization similar to previous reports by Palmaz and coworkers.[35–38] The neointimal thickness was greatest by the eighth week, and regressed to an average of 0.05 mm by the thirty-second week. Schatz concluded that this stent could be safely delivered and deployed in canine coronary arteries with acceptable long-term patency.

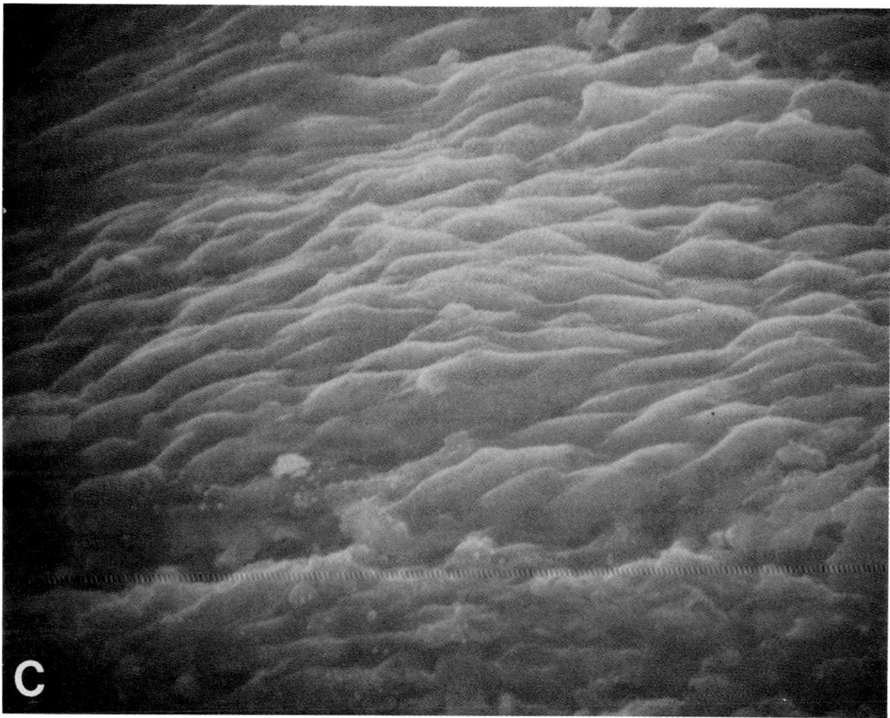

Figure 2C: *Scanning electron microscopy reveals raised immature endothelial cells.*

In an effort to improve the flexibility of the Palmaz stent, Schatz and coworkers tested an articulated version of the Palmaz stent in nine dogs.[43] Using the same anticoagulation protocol, four three-segmented stents and five two-segmented stents were placed in seven left anterior descending arteries, one intermediate, and one circumflex artery. All stented sites remained patent during 32 weeks of follow-up, and similar histopathologic results on gross and microscopic analysis were noted as in previous experiments. They concluded that the articulated stents could be safely deployed in canine coronary arteries without risk of excessive intimal hyperplasia or thrombosis.[43]

Schatz also examined the results of stenting on human cadaver coronary artery plaques. Stents were expanded in calcified coronary lesions of 15 cadaver-artery specimens within 24 hours of death.[44] Gross inspection of the stented sites revealed no signs of strut fracture. The adventitial surface of all stented segments was intact, and intimal and medial tears were noted in both control and stented sites. The intimal flaps collapsed into the vessel lumen in the control sites, and were tacked up against the arterial wall in the stented segment.

After more than 300 implants in the experimental laboratory and 3 years of follow-up in animals, the first human-stent implants in the United States

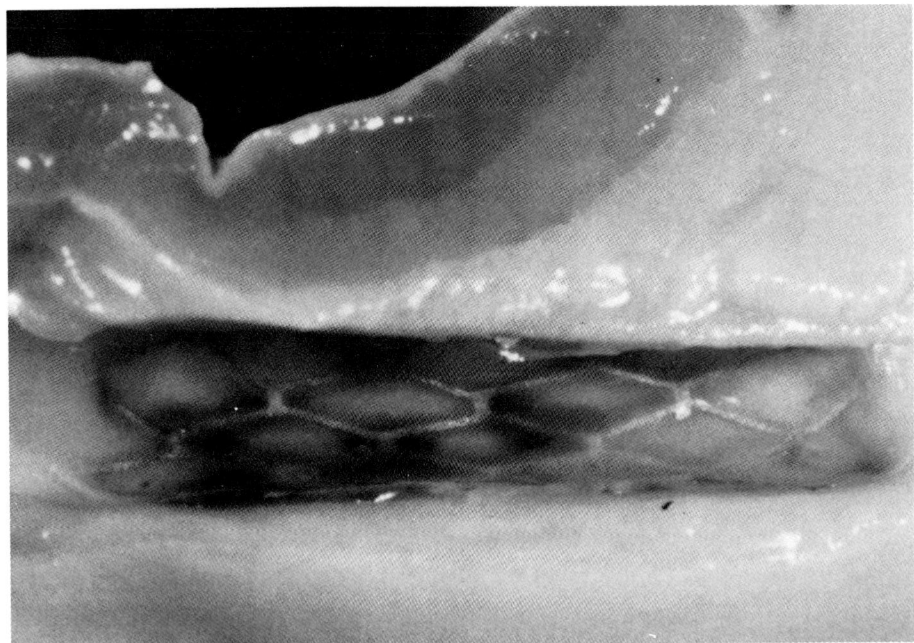

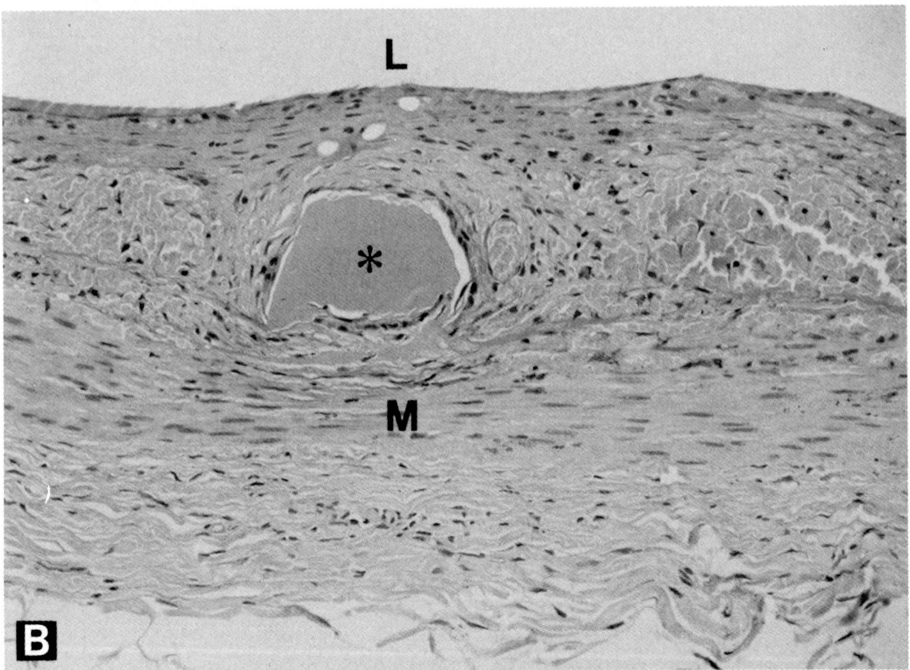

Figures 3A,3B: *At 3 weeks after experimental stent implantation,* **(A)** *gross specimen shows hemosiderin deposits, and* **(B)** *the media is compressed by the strut with thrombus replaced by myofibroblastic cells on light microscopy.*

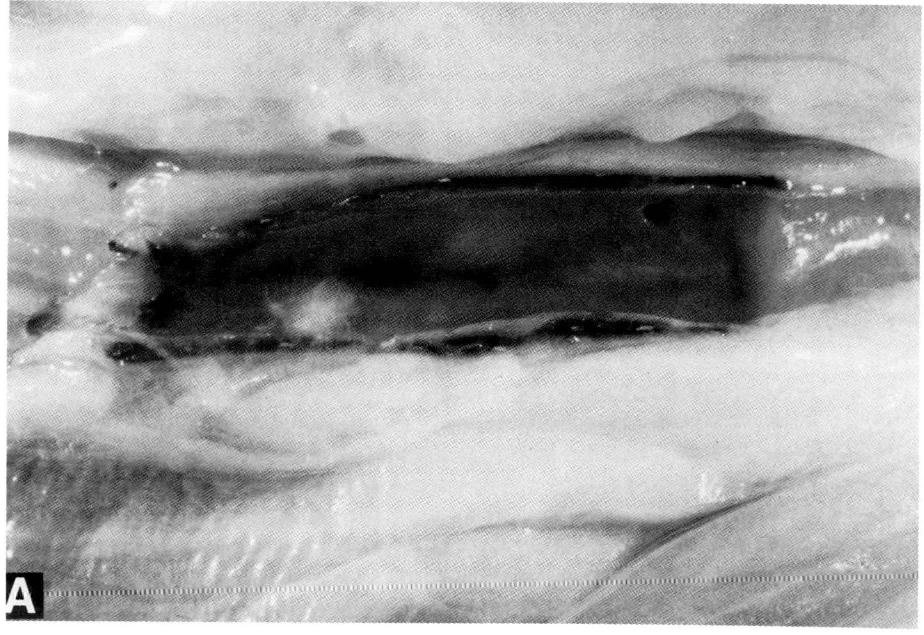

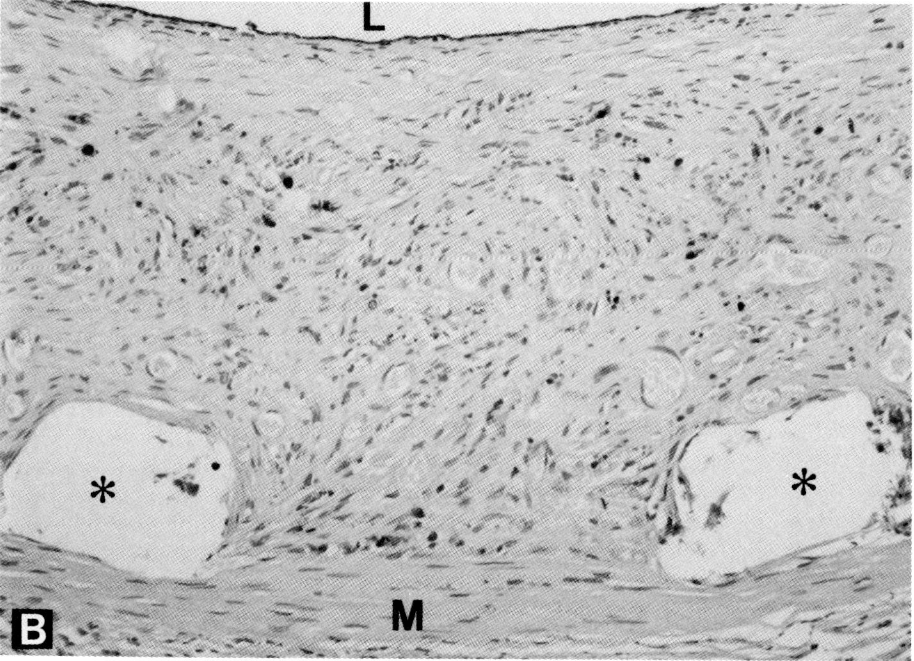

Figures 4A,4B: *By 8 weeks after experimental stent implantation,* **(A)** *the stent is covered by a thick neointima with* **(B)** *marked fibroblast proliferation on light microscopy; the neointima is thickest at this time.*

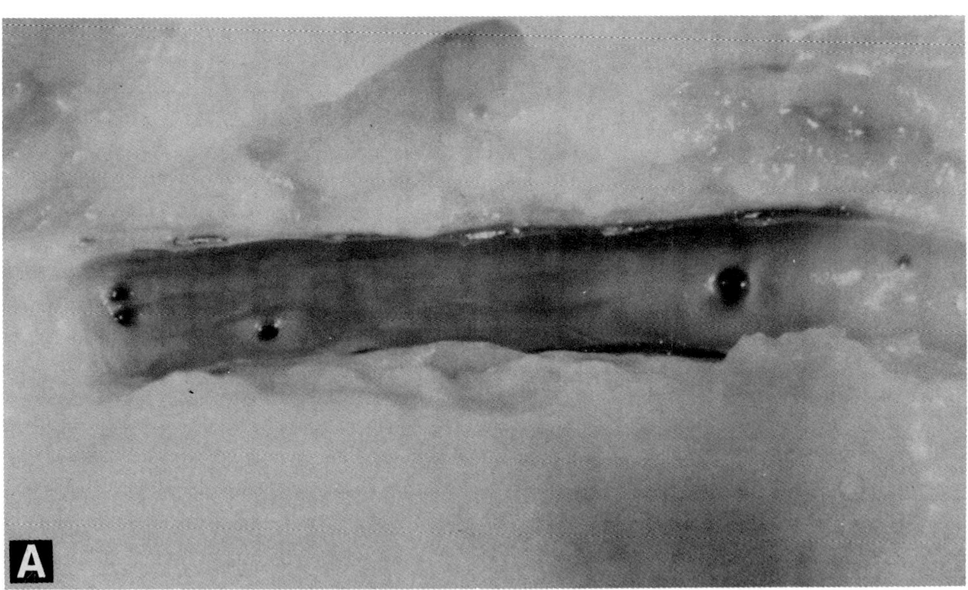

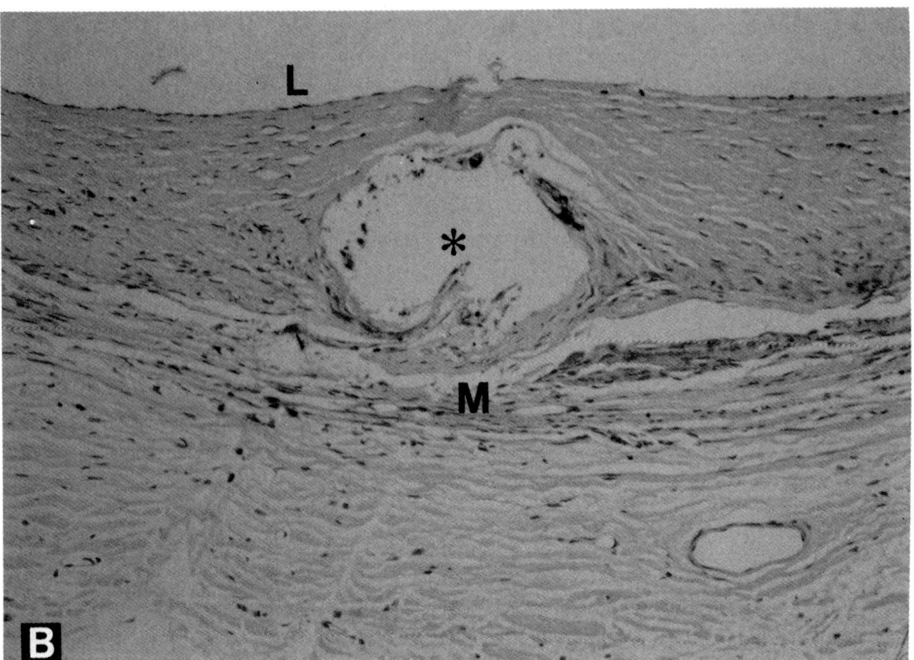

Figures 5A,5B: *By 32 weeks after experimental stent implantation,* **(A)** *the stent is easily seen through the neointima. The side branch ostia remain patent. Light microscopy* **(B)** *shows mature endothelial cells covering the sclerotic ground substance. The media becomes diffusely atrophic especially where it comes in contact with the struts.*

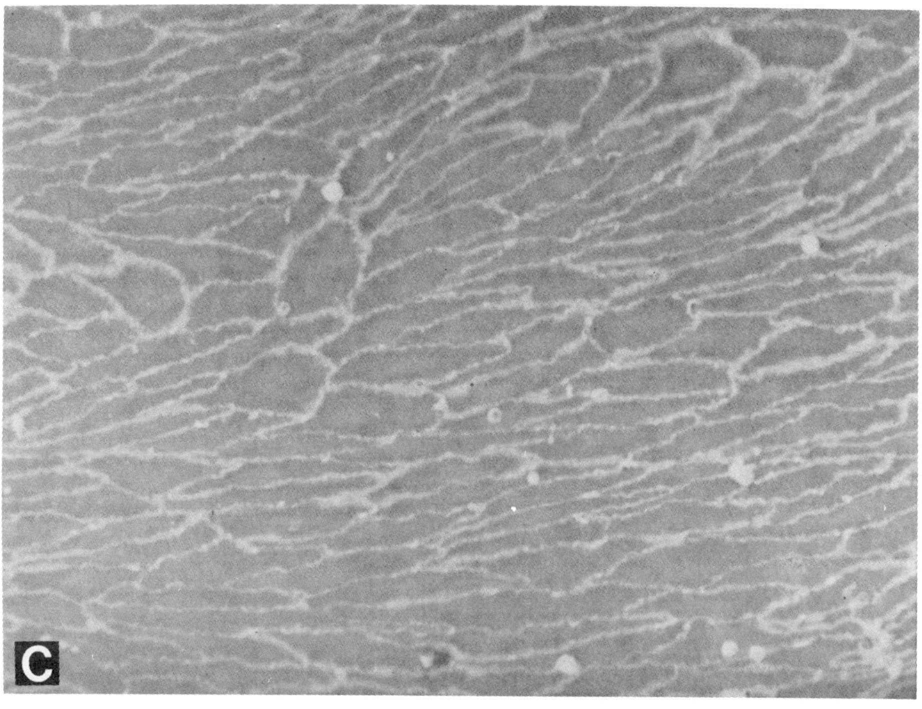

Figure 5C: *Scanning electron microscopy demonstrates that the stent is covered by mature elongated endothelial cells aligned in the direction of flow.*

and Europe, under an FDA-approved protocol, were performed by Palmaz and colleagues in May 1987.[32] The following year, Johnson and Johnson Interventional Systems received approval from the FDA to start a human coronary-stent protocol, and enrollment for this multicenter trial was started in February 1988.[45]

Current Limitations and Future Solutions

The introduction of stents into the realm of interventional cardiology has enhanced the armamentarium of the invasive cardiologist. However, there are several situations in which stenting is contraindicated or its use is limited (Table 2). Routine use is limited by the unpredictable acute and subacute thrombosis rate of 3% to 17%, despite anticoagulation and major hemorrhagic complications which may occur in 10% of patients. All current stent designs are still relatively inflexible, have rather high profiles, and are poorly visible, making deployment in tortuous vessels often difficult. Most stents are not suited for vessels smaller than 2.5 mm which are not uncommon in routine balloon angioplasty. Finally, there is a learning curve for successful deployment and prevention of complications.[46,47]

Table 2.
Current Limitations to Coronary Stent Implantation

1. Diffuse coronary disease
2. Poor vascular inflow or outflow
3. Lesion length > 15 mm
4. Extreme tortuosity of the proximal vessel
5. Vessel diameter < 2.5 mm
6. Left main disease
7. Significant thrombus at proposed target site
8. Contraindications to anticoagulation
9. Allergy to heparin, coumadin, or aspirin
10. Acute myocardial infarction

While stents appear to reduce the restenosis rate in certain subgroups of patients (i.e., discrete de novo lesions and large-caliber vessels), restenosis in vessels of coronary size has by no means been eliminated. Prolongation of hospitalization poststenting, while the patient undergoes the rather tedious but necessary adjustment of anticoagulation, will reduce the stent's appeal in today's cost-conscious medical environment.

With current devices and anticoagulation protocols, use of all stents in the setting of abrupt closure following PTCA is accompanied by high risk for subsequent stent thrombosis. Patients who receive stents under these conditions will require more intense and meticulous anticoagulation. Swars et al have published early results of provocative data that may allow for prediction of and perhaps prevention of stent thrombosis.[48]

Despite all the aforementioned shortcomings of current stent designs, one must consider that stents are relatively new devices which are still in a state of evolution. Future advances in materials and design will probably improve the profile and, hence, simplify deployment of stents in smaller and more tortuous vessels. The use of newer materials will make stents more visible and may allow more precise deployment, but will have to overcome thrombosis and metal-fatigue issues. The bonding of anticoagulant agents such as heparin[49] or antithrombin on stents may simplify the perioperative management, as well as reduce the hospital stay and hemorrhagic complications associated with current stents. The application of genetic engineering techniques may result in better thrombotic profiles or inhibition of local smooth muscle cell proliferation.[50] The development and use of biodegradable stents may result in a reduction of tissue reaction or less smooth muscle cell proliferation, once hurdles such as tensile strength and embolization are overcome.

Most of the technology that is necessary for the research and development of the "ideal" stent is currently available and under active investigation. We are hopeful that through the combined efforts of basic scientists, interventionalists, and industry, an "ideal" stent will become available in the near future.

REFERENCES

1. Dotter CT, Judkins MD: Transluminal treatment of arteriosclerotic obstruction of a new technique and a preliminary report of its application. *Circulation* 1964; 30: 654–670.
2. Dotter CT: Transluminally-placed coilspring endarterial tube grafts: long-term patency in canine popliteal artery. *Invest Radiol* 1969; 4:327–332.
3. Dotter CT, Buschmann RW, Mckinney MK, Rosch J: Transluminal expandable nitinol coil stent grafting: preliminary report. *Radiology* 1983; 147:259–260.
4. Gruentzig AR, Senning A, Siegenthaler WE: Nonoperative dilatation of coronary artery stenosis. *N Engl J Med* 1979; 301:61–68.
5. Faxon DP: Percutaneous coronary angioplasty in stable and unstable angina. *Cardiol Clin* 1991; 9:99–113.
6. Kent KM: Coronary angioplasty: a decade of experience. *N Engl J Med* 1987; 316: 1148–1150.
7. Detre K, Holubkov R, Kelsey S, Cowley MJ, Kent K, Williams D, Myler R, Faxon D, Holmes D Jr, Bourassa M, Block P, Gosselin A, Bentivoglio L, Leatherman L, Dorros G, King S, Galichia J, Al-Bassam M, Leon M, Robertson T, Passamani E, and the coinvestigators of the National Heart, Lung, and Blood Institute's Percutaneous Transluminal Coronary Angioplasty Registry: Percutaneous transluminal coronary angioplasty in 1985–1986 and 1977–1981. *N Engl J Med* 1988; 318:265–270.
8. Cragg A, Lund G, Rysavy J, Castaneda F, Castaneda-Zuniga W, Amplatz K: Nonsurgical placement of arterial endoprostheses: a new technique using nitinol wire. *Radiology* 1983; 147:261–263.
9. Maass D, Zllikofer CL, Largiader F, Senning A: Radiological follow-up of transluminally inserted vascular endoprostheses: an experimental study using expanding spirals. *Radiology* 1984; 152:659–663.
10. Wright KC, Wallace S, Charnsangavej C, Carrasco CH, Gianturco C: Percutaneous endovascular stents: an experimental evaluation. *Radiology* 1982; 156:69–72.
11. Palmaz JC, Sibbitt RR, Reuter ST, Tio FO, Rice WJ: Expandable intraluminal graft: a preliminary study. *Radiology* 1985; 156:73–77.
12. Palmaz JC, Windeler SAM, Garcia FM, Tio FO, Sibbitt RR, Reuter SR: Atherosclerotic rabbit aortas: expandable intraluminal grafting. *Radiology* 1986; 16O: 723–726.
13. Palmaz JC, Schatz RA, Richter G, Gardiner G, Becker G, Garcia O: Intraluminal stenting of iliac artery stenosis: preliminary report of a multicenter trial. *Circulation* 1988; 78(suppl II):II-415. Abstract.
14. Detre K, Holmes D, Holubkov R, Cowley MJ, Bourassa M, Faxon D, Dorros G, Bentivoglio L, Kent K, Myler R: Incidence and consequences of periprocedural occlusion: the 1985–1986 NHLBI percutaneous transluminal coronary angioplasty registry. *Circulation* 1990; 82:739–750.
15. Muller DWM, Ellis SG: Advances in coronary angioplasty: endovascular stents. *Coronary Artery Disease* 1990; 1:438–448.
16. King SB: Vascular stents and atherosclerosis. *Circulation* 1989; 79:460–462.
17. Holmes DR, Vlietstra RE, Smith HC, Vetrovec G, Kent KM, Cowley MJ, Faxon DP, Gruentzig AR, Kelsey SF, Detre KM, Van Raden MJ, Mock MB: Restenosis after PTCA: a report from the PTCA registry of the National Heart, Lung, and Blood Institute. *Am J Cardiol* 1984; 53:77C-81C.
18. Gruentzig AR, King SB, Schlumpf M, Siegenthaler W: Long-term follow-up after percutaneous transluminal coronary angioplasty: The early Zurich experience. *N Engl J Med* 1987; 316:1127–1132.
19. Serruys PW, Luijten KJ, Beatt KJ, Geuskens BR, DeFeyter PJ, Van Den Brand M, Reiber JHC, Ten Kate HJ, Van Es GA, Hugenholtz PG: Incidence of restenosis after successful coronary angioplasty: a time-related phenomenon: a quantitative

angiographic study in 342 consecutive patients at 1, 2, 3, and 4 months. *Circulation* 1988; 77:361–371.
20. Webb JG, Myler RK, Shaw RE, Anwar A, Mayo JR, Murphy MC, Cumberland DC, Stertzer SH: Coronary angioplasty after coronary bypass surgery: initial results and late outcome in 422 patients. *J Am Coll Cardiol* 1990; 16:812–820.
21. Hirshfeld JW, Schwartz JS, Jugo R, Macdonald RG, Goldberg S, Savage MP, Bass TA, Vetrovec G, Cowley M, Taussig AS, Whitworth HB, Margolis JR, Hill JA, Pepine CJ and the M-HEART Investigators: Restenosis after coronary angioplasty: a multivariate statistical model to relate lesion and procedure variables to restenosis. *J Am Coll Cardiol* 1991; 18:647–656.
22. Nobuyoshi M, Kimura T, Nosaka H, Mioka S, Ueno K, Yokoi H, Hamasaki N, Horiuchi H, Ohishi H: Restenosis after successful percutaneous transluminal coronary angioplasty: serial angiographic follow-up of 229 patients. *J Am Coll Cardiol* 1988; 12:616–623.
23. Wigns W, Serruys PW, Reiber JHC: Early detection of restenosis after successful percutaneous transluminal coronary angioplasty by execise-redistribution thallium scintigraphy. *Am J Cardiol* 1985; 55:357–361.
24. Powelson S, Roubin G, Whitworth H, Gruentzig A: Incidence of early restenosis after successful percutaneous transluminal coronary angioplasty. *J Am Coll Cardiol* 1986; 7:63A. Abstract.
25. Rensing BJ, Hermans WRM, Beatt KJ, Laarman GJ, Suryapranata H, Van Den Brand M, DeFeyter PJ, Serruys PW: Quantitative angiographic assessment of elastic recoil after percutaneous transluminal coronary angioplasty. *Am J Cardiol* 1990; 66:1039–1044.
26. Beatt KJ, Bertrand M, Puel J, Richards T, Serruys PW, Sigwart U: Additional improvement in vessel lumen in the first 24 hours after stent implantation due to radial dilating force. *J Am Coll Cardiol* 1989; 13:224A. Abstract.
27. Raizner AE, Minor ST, Siegel CO, Woolbert SP, Abukhalil JM, Roberts MA: Dimensional stability of the Gianturco-Roubin balloon expandable stent assessed by quantitative coronary angiography. *J Am Coll Cardiol* 1991; 17:301A. Abstract.
28. Ku DN, Giddens DP, Farins CK, Glagov S : Pulsatile flow and atherosclerosis in human carotid bifurcation: positive correlation between plaque and low and oscillating shear stress. *Arteriosclerosis* 1985; 5:292–302.
29. Zarins CK, Bomgerger RA, Glagov S: Local effects of stenoses: increased flow velocity inhibits atherogenesis. *Circulation* 1991; (suppl II)Il-221-II-227.
30. Palmaz JC: Balloon-expandable intravascular stent. *Am J Radiol* 1988; 150: 1263–69.
31. Zollikofer CL, Largiader I, Bruhlmann WF, Uhlschmid GK, Marty AH: Endovascular stenting of veins and grafts: preliminary clinical experience. *Radiology* 1988; 167:707–712.
32. Schatz RA: A view of vascular stents. *Circulation* 1989; 79:445–457.
33. Rousseau H, Puel J, Joffre F, Sigwart U, Duboucher C, Imbert C, Knight C, Kropf L, Wallsten H: Self-expanding endovascular prosthesis: an experimental study. *Radiology* 1987; 164:709.
34. Sigwart U, Puel J, Mirkovitch V, Joffre F, Kappenberger L: Intravascular stents to prevent occlusion and restenosis after transluminal angioplasty. *N Engl J Med* 1987; 316:701–706.
35. Palmaz JC, Sibbitt M;, Reuter SR, Tio FO, Rice WJ: Expandable intraluminal graft: preliminary study. *Radiology* 1985; 156:73–77.
36. Palmaz JC, Windelar S, Garcia F, Tio FO, Sibbitt RR, Reuter SR: Atherosclerotic rabbit aortas: expandable intraluminal grafting. *Radiology* 1986; 160:723–726.
37. Palmaz JC, Sibbitt RR, Tio FO, Reuter SR, Peters JE, Garcia F: Expandable intraluminal vascular graft: a feasibility study. *Surgery* 1985; 99:199–205.
38. Palmaz JC, Koopp DT, Hayashi H, Schatz R, Hunter G, Tio FO, Garcia O, Alvarado

R, Rees C, Thomas SC: Normal and stenotic renal arteries: experimental balloon-expandable intraluminal stenting. *Radiology* 1987; 164:705–708.

39. Schatz RA, Palmaz JC: Intravascular stents for angioplasty. *Cardiology* 1987; 27–31.
40. Schatz RA, Palmaz JC: Balloon expandable intravascular stents (BEIS) in human coronary arteries: report of initial experience. *Circulation* 1988; 78(suppl II):II-1625. Abstract.
41. Baim DS, Bailey S, Curry C, Walker C, Schatz RA: Improved success and safety of Palmaz-Schatz coronary stenting with a new delivery system. *Circulation* 1990; 82(suppl III):III-657. Abstract.
42. Palmaz JC, Garcia 0, Kopp DB, et al: Balloon-expandable intra-arterial stents: effect of antithrombotic medication on thrombus formation. In: Seither C, Seyferth W, eds. *Pros and Cons in PTA and Auxiliary Methods*. Berlin: Springer-Verlag, 1989.
43. Schatz RA, Palmaz JC, Tio F, Garcia 0: Report of a new articulated balloon expandable intravascular stent. *Circulation* 1988; 78(suppl II):449. Abstract.
44. Schatz RA, Tio FO, Palmaz JC: Balloon expandable intravascular stents in diseased human cadaver coronary arteries. *Circulation* 1987; 76(suppl IV):IV-26.
45. Schatz RA, Baim DS, Leon M, Ellis SG, Goldberg S, Hirshfeld JW, Cleman MW, Cabin HS, Walker C, Stagg J, Buchbinder M, Tierstein PS, Topol EJ, Savage M, Perez JA, Curry RC, Whitworth H, Sousa JE, Tio FO, Almagor Y, Ponder R, Penn IM, Leonard B, Levine SL, Fish RD, Palmaz JC: Clinical experience with the Palmaz-Schatz coronary stent: initial results of a multicenter study. *Circulation* 1991; 83:148–161.
46. Sigwart U, Urban P, Sadeghi H, Kappenberger L: Implantation of 100 coronary artery stents: learning curve for the incidence of acute early complication. *J Am Coll Cardiol* 1989; 13:107A. Abstract.
47. Roubin GS, Agrawal S, Dean LS, Barley WA, Garrahy P, Cavender J, Macender P, Carrion : What are the predictors of acute complications following coronary artery stenting?: single institutional experience. *J Am Coll Cardiol* 1991; 17:281A. Abstract.
48. Swars H, Hafner G, Erbel R, Ehrenthal W, Rupprecht HJ, Prellwitz W, Meyer J: Prothrombin fragment F1 + 2 predicts acute occlusion after intracoronary stenting. *J Am Coll Cardiol* 1991; 17:302A. Abstract.
49. Hearn JA, Robinson KA, Roubin GS: In-vitro thrombus formation of stent wires: role of metallic composition and heparin coating. *J Am Coll Cardiol* 1991; 17:302A. Abstract.
50. Dichek DA, Neville RF, Zwiebel JA, Freeman SM, Leon MB, Anderson WF: Seeding of intravascular stents with genetically engineered endothelial cells. *Circulation* 1989; 80:1347–1353.

II

Stent Insertion

CHAPTER 2

Stent Deployment:
Technical Considerations

John W. Hirshfeld Jr.
Howard C. Herrmann

Coronary stenting is a technically demanding procedure which requires, as a prerequisite, considerable knowledge, skill, and experience in conventional coronary angioplasty. Although the techniques of stent deployment in the coronary circulation are similar to conventional coronary angioplasty, they are more demanding, the procedure and the instruments are less forgiving, and there are a number of unique considerations and difficulties. Several fundamental differences between the two procedures must be thoroughly understood if one is to succeed and avoid complications.

Description of the Stent-Delivery System

The Role of the Stent-Delivery System

The history of the design evolution of the Palmaz-Schatz stent and the stent-delivery system is covered in Chapter 1. The early clinical experience with stenting involved the delivery of an exposed stent after hand-crimping it onto a conventional angioplasty balloon catheter.

It rapidly became apparent that this approach had several important shortcomings which contributed to failed delivery attempts and, more importantly, embolization of undeployed stents. The integrity of the delivery system depended upon the security of the crimp that was performed by the operator at the time of the procedure. The potential for variation of crimp security constituted a potential cause for delivery failure. Tracking curves in the target vessel requires flexing of the stent. This may cause the tips of the stent-end struts to

From: Herrmann HC, Hirshfeld JW, eds. *Clinical Use of the Palmaz-Schatz Intracoronary Stent.* Futura Publishing Company, Inc., Mount Kisco, NY, © 1993.

bend away from their crimped position and allow them to snag on the wall of the target vessel, preventing the stent from reaching the target site. In the event of a failed delivery attempt, withdrawal of the delivery catheter and stent not protected by a sheath almost invariably strips the stent off the delivery catheter, causing embolization.[1] Although there have been no adverse consequences of peripheral stent embolization, this is obviously an undesirable event.

Design of the Stent-Delivery System

The currently used stent-delivery system is illustrated in Figure 1. The basic concept behind the system is a retractable sheath that covers the stent and the stent-delivery balloon assembly during delivery to the target site. It was developed to address the problems of delivery failure and embolization as described above. It trades the complexity, decreased trackability, and larger

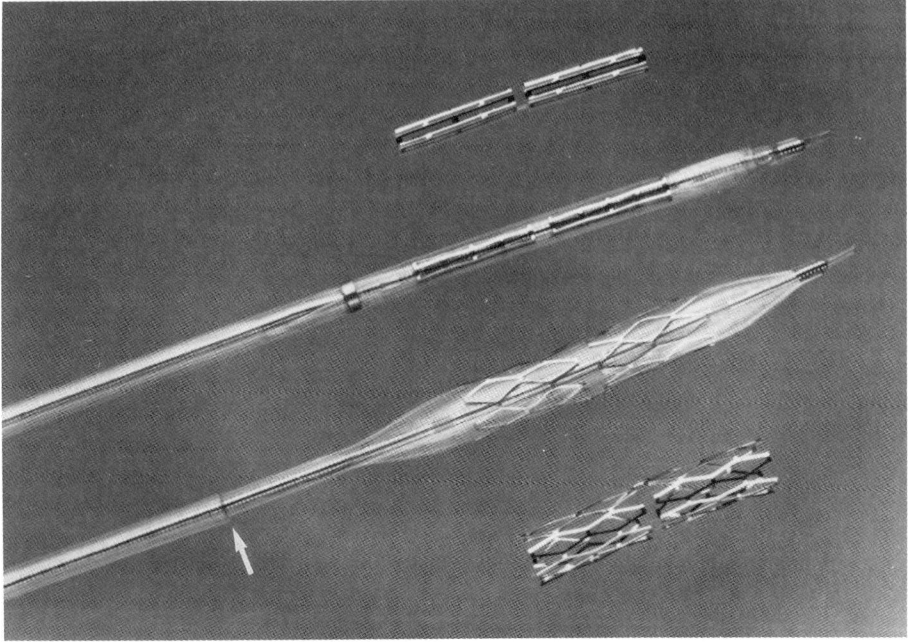

Figure 1: *The currently available stent-delivery system. It consists of a specifically designed stent-delivery balloon catheter which has two gold markers 18 mm apart, an articulated coronary-stent factory-crimped onto the balloon catheter between the two markers, and a 4.8-F nylon sheath (arrow) which has a platinum marker located 3 cm proximal to its tip. The delivery catheter and stent assembly are mounted inside the sheath. The purpose of the sheath marker (which could not be located at the tip of the sheath because it adversely affected the sheath's profile) is to disclose the relationship between the sheath and the stent-delivery catheter.*

profile of the sheath system for the security of being able to abort a failed delivery procedure without embolizing the stent, and a reduced likelihood of snagging on the target vessel. With the introduction of the sheath-delivery system, delivery success has improved, and embolization has been virtually eliminated.[2]

The stent-delivery system consists of a stent mounted on the balloon of a stent-delivery catheter contained within a specially designed sheath. The balloon is designed so that it wings at its tips. This design, which would be undesirable for a conventional angioplasty catheter, enhances the security of the crimp of the stent onto the balloon. The balloon material is compliant and, at a rated-burst pressure of approximately 6 atmosphere (ATM), not particularly strong. The sheath is made of nylon. This material was chosen from a large number of candidate materials for its ability to flex and, thus, not degrade trackability, yet have sufficient axial strength at a small-wall thickness so that it would retract reliably to expose the stent when the delivery system was in position.

The sheath has a radiopaque marker band attached 3 cm from the tip which is necessary to disclose the relationship of the sheath to the stent-delivery catheter. The marker band is located proximally so that it does not increase the diameter of the sheath tip. Another important feature is that the marker is actually mounted inside the sheath. This feature, which reduces profile, has an important consequence. The inside diameter of the sheath at the marker band is less than the diameter of the crimped stent. If the sheath is advanced past the tip of the stent-delivery catheter, it may strip the stent off the balloon catheter, potentially causing embolization. The security of the relationship between the sheath and the balloon catheter is maintained by locking the Touhy-Borst washer (Advanced Cardiovascular Systems, Temecula, CA) of the sheath's Y-connector. Therefore, when the stent-delivery system is to be manipulated as a unit, this washer must be tight.

Differences Between Conventional Balloon Angioplasty and Stent Implantation

Delivery Difficulties

The current (1992) version of the stent-delivery system, which is described and illustrated above, is considerably more difficult to deliver to a target site than the current conventional angioplasty balloons, for a variety of reasons.

1. The stent-delivery system's diameter is 4.8F (.063 inches). This is substantially larger than conventional angioplasty balloons which range between 2.5F and 3.0 F(.032 to .039 inches). Consequently, it must be delivered through a guide catheter with a minimum diameter of .078 inches. Virtually all currently available 8F-guide catheters (but no 7F-catheters) meet this specification. Because of its diameter, the system takes up a considerable amount of space within the guide catheter and the coronary vessel. This impairs the abil-

ity to measure pressure and inject a contrast agent through the guide catheter. The contrast-agent injection problem is important because good visualization of the target site is critical for accurate deployment. Not only is it difficult to inject the contrast agent through the guide catheter at a sufficiently rapid rate, but the stent-delivery system, because of its large diameter, frequently obstructs the vessel to a degree that impairs target-site visualization and provokes substantial ischemia. This can complicate the task of stent delivery and deployment because the ischemia may require operators to work rapidly.

2. The profile and taper of the stent-delivery system is considerably blunter than that of conventional angioplasty balloon catheters. This can cause difficulty in crossing either the target stenosis or a noncritically stenosed more proximal portion of the target vessel.

3. The system is substantially less trackable than a conventional angioplasty balloon catheter. The system consists of three coaxial devices; the stent-delivery balloon catheter, the stent itself, and the external sheath. The stent itself consists of two inflexible 7-mm segments, and can flex at the central articulation site only. Each of these devices contributes to a degradation of the trackability of the entire assembly.

4. In its current version, the stent-delivery system provides approximately 20 cm of useable length, depending on the type of Y-connector used. This is less than that provided by a conventional balloon catheter.

Thus, the stent-delivery system's bulk, blunt profile, and poor trackability increase the demands on the operator when endeavoring to deliver a stent to a target site. These limitations indicate that delivery of a stent to a target site in a tortuous or small-diameter vessel may be difficult, if not impossible. The limitations also place greater demands for guide-catheter support in order to be able to advance the stent-delivery system against resistance. Guide-catheter selection and positioning thus becomes an important consideration. Catheters should be selected for their ability to provide backup support and to align accurately with the proximal portion of the target coronary artery.

Requirement for Accurate Deployment

Once deployed, a stent cannot be repositioned. Unlike conventional balloon angioplasty when a second properly positioned inflation can be performed if the initial balloon inflation is not perfectly positioned with respect to the lesion, there is only one chance to place a stent correctly.

Positioning Considerations

There are a number of issues to consider when deciding exactly where to deploy a stent. Centering a stent with respect to the target lesion is not always the ideal strategy for several reasons.

1. It is undesirable to place a stent across a major side branch. Although such side branches virtually always remain patent because blood can flow through the gaps between the stent struts,[3] it is possible that the stent may partially impair flow into the vessel. A more important consideration is that placing a stent across a major side branch places the branch in "stent jail," precluding future access to that branch with any angioplasty device.

2. If multiple tandem stents are to be placed, the degree of overlap should be minimized, since overlap may increase the tissue reaction at that area,[4] and increase the rate of restenosis.[5] Thus, if an anatomical situation calls for the placement of multiple tandem stents, the location of any one stent will dictate the location of the adjacent stents. For example, if the most proximal of a group of tandem stents would be forced to protrude out of a coronary orifice, the most distal stent of the group should be placed more distally to allow the most proximal stent to be appropriately positioned.

3. Once a stent has been placed, it may not be possible to place another stent more distally in the vessel because of snagging of the stent-delivery system on the already deployed stent. Consequently, if multiple stents are to be placed, the plan for stent delivery should always involve placing the most distal stent first and working proximally.

4. Occasionally, the stent's 1-mm gap at the center articulation of the stent leaves a portion of a lesion inadequately supported. Thus, particularly with very short discrete lesions, it may be preferable to place the stent several millimeters off center with respect to the lesion.

Considerations in Lesion Selection

Not all coronary lesions are suitable for stenting. In considering a candidate lesion for stenting, it is important to examine whether it is feasible to deliver a stent to the target site, and how well the stent, once delivered, will perform. These important considerations may be divided into characteristics of the target vessel proximal to the stent-deployment site and the characteristics of the target lesion.

The tortuosity, size, degree of atherosclerotic narrowing of the target vessel proximal to the lesion, and the type of guide-catheter fit which can be achieved influence the likelihood that a stent can be successfully delivered to and deployed at the target site. The size of the vessel at the site of stent deployment has an important influence on the likelihood of restenosis, with vessels smaller than 3.0 mm having a greater restenosis rate[5] (see Chapter 11). The presence of important side branches close to the target lesion may make it less suitable for stenting. Lesions which are very close or in the left main coronary bifurcation may be undesirable if the proximal portion of the stent must protrude into the left main artery, although stenting in this location has been successfully accomplished.[6] Similarly, stents placed close to the orifice of a coronary artery or a vein graft are vulnerable to damage by the tip of the guide catheter or may, if not properly positioned, protrude into the aorta.

Stenting has been less effective in long, diffuse lesions. Such lesions often require multiple overlapping stents to cover their entire length, and have had an increased restenosis rate.[5] However, characteristics such as eccentricity, geometric complexity, location on a bend, and calcification (characteristics which are associated with decreased success rates for conventional angioplasty) do not appear to undermine the success of stenting.

Pharmacologic Management

In conventional angioplasty, antithrombotic therapy is the cornerstone of pharmacologic management. However, because stenting involves implantation of a potentially prothrombotic device into an area of fresh vascular injury, assiduous attention to the details of antithrombotic therapy is particularly important. Careful monitoring of the degree of anticoagulation during the periprocedural period is essential because one must walk a narrow tightrope between inadequate antithrombotic therapy (predisposing to stent thrombosis) and excessive anticoagulation (increasing the likelihood of bleeding and vascular entry site complications). The antithrombotic program currently recommended is summarized in Table 1, and has been developed through a combina-

Table 1.
Antithrombotic Therapy for Stent Implantation

Preprocedure
- Aspirin 325 mg per day including the day of the procedure.
- Dipyridamole 75 mg T.I.D. beginning at least the evening before the procedure.
- Warfarin 10 mg the evening before the procedure.
- 10% low-molecular weight Dextran I.V. at 100 ml/h beginning 4 h before the procedure.

Intraprocedure
- Continue 10% low-molecular weight dextran I.V. at 50 ml/h.
- Heparin 10,000 U I.V. with supplementation as needed to maintain activated clotting time greater than 350 s through the procedure.

Early Postprocedure
- Initially do not continue heparin unless plans are to delay catheter removal. Restart heparin 2 hours following catheter removal without a bolus. Adjust infusion rate to achieve a PTT between 60 s and 90 s.
- Continue 10% low-molecular weight dextran at 50 ml/h until a total dose of 1000 mL has been administered.
- Continue aspirin and dipyridamole.
- Warfarin 10 mg the evening following the procedure.

Late Postprocedure
- Continue warfarin to achieve PT 16.0–18.0 (INR 2.0–3.0). Maintain PT in that range for 30 days postimplantation.
- Continue I.V. heparin until PT is greater than 16.0 for 24 h.
- Continue aspirin indefinitely.
- Continue dipyridamole for 4 m.

tion of animal studies, clinical intuition, and clinical experience. The basis of this regimen is reviewed in Chapter 3.

Preprocedural Preparation

Antiplatelet therapy should be started prior to the procedure. It should include aspirin, 325 mg per day including the day of the procedure, and dipyridamole, 75 mg T.I.D beginning at least the day before the procedure. Since warfarin anticoagulation is required following the procedure, it may be begun with a dose of 10 mg the evening before. A 10% low-molecular weight dextran solution infusion should begin 4 hours prior to the procedure at an infusion rate of 100 mL per hour. The goal is to achieve a total delivered dose of 500 mL by the time the stent is actually deployed.

Intraprocedural Management

The dextran infusion is continued at 50 mL per hour. Standard angioplasty heparin anticoagulation is employed, with the dose adjusted by the results of the activated clotting time (ACT). A minimum ACT of 350 seconds should be achieved. At the conclusion of the procedure, the ACT should be checked and additional heparin given, if necessary, to maintain this minimum value.

Early Postprocedural Management

Following stent deployment, provided a satisfactory angiographic result with no evidence of thrombus within the stent has been achieved, heparin is not continued, and catheters are removed when the ACT falls below 175 seconds (usually 4 to 6 hours following the implantation). During this period, the dextran infusion is continued at a rate of 50 ml per hour until a total dose of 1000 mL has been administered. Heparin is restarted without a bolus, 2 hours after catheter removal at an infusion rate sufficient to maintain a partial thromboplastin time between 60 and 90 seconds. Warfarin is administered and the heparin infusion is continued until the prothrombin time has been greater than 16 seconds (international normalized ratio [INR] $>$ 2.0) for at least 24 hours.

Late Postprocedural Management

Warfarin therapy to maintain the prothrombin time between 16.0 seconds and 18.0 seconds (INR between 2.0 and 3.0) is continued for 1 month following stent deployment. By the time the stent has been implanted for 1 month, it is fully coated with neointima and is no longer at risk of thrombosis (see Chapter 1). Aspirin is continued indefinitely. Dipyridamole is continued for 4 months.

Deployment Technique

General Requirements

Guide Catheters

The stent-delivery system is compatible with all currently used guide-catheter curves, and can be used with any commercially available guide catheter with a lumen diameter of at least .078 inches. Larger catheters (e.g., 9F) may be helpful in an operator's early experience to improve backup support and visualization.

Guidewires

The stent-delivery system will accept a maximum guidewire diameter of .014 inches. Some commercially available 300-cm guidewires, which are listed as .014 inches have .016-inch proximal segments and should not be used. It is compatible with guidewire-extension systems provided that no portion of the system exceeds .014 inches in diameter. However, because of the tightness of the tolerances, any kink in the guidewire or any imperfection of the joint between the guidewire and its extension will cause unacceptable impairment of guidewire movement. The stent-delivery system has not been tested yet with balloon-guidewire exchange devices such as the Sci-Med "Trapper" (SciMed Life Systems, Inc., Maple Grove, MN). However, it is likely that such a device could not be used with a .078-inch lumen-guide catheter and that a guide-catheter diameter of at least .091 inches would probably be required.

Y-Connectors

The Y-connector used to introduce the stent-delivery system into the guide catheter must be capable of accepting a .065-inch diameter instrument. Currently, several such devices are commercially available.

Radiological Considerations

The requirements for the radiological projections used for stent deployment are similar to but somewhat more stringent than those used for conventional angioplasty. The radiological projection should delineate the location of the proximal and distal ends of the target lesion and the locations of any major nearby branches. Careful attention should be paid to the existence of any landmarks such as branches or surgical clips which will assist in identifying the location of the target lesion and determining the relationship of the stent delivery system to it during deployment.

Goals for Stent Deployment

The goal of stenting should be to achieve complete expansion of the stent with uniform contact of all its portions with the vascular wall, and a final percent stenosis of zero or better. If the stent is not uniformly expanded, the gaps between the partially expanded stent and the vessel wall are sites where blood stasis and thrombosis may occur. The goal of overexpansion to achieve a percent stenosis of less than zero is to accommodate the inevitable subsequent loss of lumen dimension consequent to neointimal ingrowth. The enhanced lumen dimension that can be achieved by stenting is probably the mechanism of whatever favorable impact stenting may have on restenosis. In contrast to conventional coronary angioplasty in which overexpansion of the target site is hazardous, the presence of the stent protects against dissection and supports the target site at a larger dimension.

Preparation of the Stent-Delivery System

The stent-delivery system is described above. It is designed to be "doctor proof" so that minimal operator preparation is required. However, several aspects of its assembly should be checked and adjusted prior to use.

1. The stent-delivery system is shipped assembled, with the stent-delivery catheter and the stent within the stent-delivery sheath and Y-connector. Because this system is assembled sterilized, the shaft of the stent-delivery catheter frequently adheres to the washer of the sheath's Y-connector Tuohy-Borst valve. This adhesion should be broken and free movement of the stent-delivery catheter within the sheath should be assured prior to introducing the system into the patient.

2. The relationship of the stent-delivery catheter to the tip of the sheath is critical to the tracking performance of the system. This relationship is crudely adjusted at the factory, but almost always requires fine tuning before the device is introduced into the patient. The tip of the stent-delivery balloon catheter can serve as an obturator to facilitate the passage of the blunt and bulky sheath through tortuous vascular segments. Therefore, the tip of the balloon catheter should protrude from the sheath as far as possible without exposing the stent. Because the shaft of the balloon catheter is somewhat compressible longitudinally, the sheath should initially be adjusted so that the distal 2 mm of the stent protrudes past the tip of the sheath when force is not applied to the tip of the catheter. Application of force to the tip of the catheter will push it back so that the stent is just inside the sheath and it will not be exposed when the delivery system is advanced against resistance. Once this relationship is achieved, it must be maintained by tightly locking the washer of the Y-connector onto the stent-delivery catheter. The inner member of the stent-delivery catheter is reinforced with a helical wire winding, which gives it considerable radial strength to resist collapse by the washer. In extreme circumstances, if

the Touhy-Borst washer is not tightened sufficiently, the sheath may be forced past the tip of the delivery catheter during attempts to advance it. Because the internal diameter of the sheath at the location of the marker is less than the diameter of the crimped stent, this will strip the stent off the balloon tip and may allow an unexpanded stent to embolize within the coronary vessel.

3. The lumens of the sheath and the stent-delivery balloon should be primed with heparinized saline. The sideport of the sheath Y-connector should be stopcocked. In general, a Y-connector is not needed for the stent-delivery balloon because the fit between the central lumen of the balloon and the .014-inch guidewire is very tight, and the system is generally not in the patient for more than a few minutes.

4. The balloon of the stent-delivery catheter should not be prepared until the stent has been delivered to the target site, the sheath has been retracted, and the position of the stent-delivery catheter has been finely adjusted to the position for deployment. This is because the security of the crimp of the stent on the balloon is diminished once vacuum is applied to the balloon to prepare it. Once the balloon has been evacuated, movement of the balloon within the coronary vessel is more likely to strip off the stent.

Delivery Technique

The basic steps in the delivery process are a predilation of the target lesion (if necessary) to enable the bulky stent-delivery system to reach the target site, delivery of the stent-delivery system to the target site, exposure and deployment of the stent, and final expansion of the stent to the desired diameter. The entire process often involves several catheter exchanges. Thus, in a planned elective stent deployment it is best to conduct the entire procedure using a 300 cm .014-inch guidewire. This wire is compatible with all devices which may be needed, and allows the multiple catheter exchanges required without wire exchanges or extensions.

The guide catheter should be selected according to the above outlined requirements. Given the greater difficulty of delivering the stent-delivery system to the target site, the most appropriate guide-catheter curve is that which will provide the best backup support. For example, a lesion in the left circumflex coronary artery, which could be successfully crossed by a low-profile balloon catheter using a Judkins-curve guide catheter may require the additional backup support and better alignment furnished by an Amplatz curve. In general, guide catheters with proximal side holes should be avoided. One of the major difficulties of stent deployment is ascertaining the exact location of the stent prior to expansion. Contrast-agent delivery into the target vessel is impaired by the large diameter of the stent-delivery system which interferes both with injection through the guide catheter and with flow into the target vessel. This problem is accentuated if the guide catheter has proximal side holes.

The basic delivery technique is colloquially referred to as "the under-over technique." This consists of a small-diameter predilation with a conventional balloon, followed by deployment of the stent. The procedure is finished by further expansion of the stent to a diameter equal to or greater than the diameter of the adjacent vessel with a high-pressure balloon. The steps of stent delivery, deployment, and finishing are illustrated in Figures 2 through 8. Baseline angiography (Fig. 2) should accurately delineate the above described anatomical relationships. The first step is to pass a 300-cm .014-inch guidewire across the stenosis. Predilation can be performed with an undersized balloon, but it is not always necessary if the target lesion is soft or if it has a sufficient lumen diameter to allow the stent-delivery system to cross it. The speculative rationale for predilation with an undersized balloon is that it is preferable not to produce dissection flaps prior to stent deployment. A flap might impair the delivery of the stent-delivery system or might increase the target site's thrombogenicity.

Once the target site is ready to receive the stent, the predilating catheter is removed, leaving the guidewire in position across the stenosis. The stent-delivery system is prepared as described above and introduced onto the guidewire, but the balloon is not evacuated. Because of the tight fit between the stent-delivery balloon catheter and the guidewire, it is essential that the external portion of the guidewire be wiped thoroughly several times following balloon-catheter withdrawal. The distal tip of the stent-delivery system is introduced into the Tuohy-Borst Y-connector on the guide catheter and advanced to the distal tip of the guide catheter. The guide-catheter position is adjusted to provide optimal backup support, and the stent-delivery system is advanced into the target vessel and to the target site (Fig. 3). During positioning of the stent-delivery system within the target vessel and lesion, careful attention must be paid to the relationship between the stent-delivery catheter and the sheath as disclosed by the two markers on the balloon and the more proximal marker on the sheath. The stent itself is faintly visible as a slight increase in the radiographical density between the two balloon markers (Fig. 3). This should be observed because it is the only way that the operator can determine whether the stent has shifted its position on the delivery balloon.

Once the target site is reached, the correct positioning of the stent within the target site is verified, and the sheath is retracted to expose the stent. The retraction is accomplished by simultaneously advancing the stent-delivery catheter and withdrawing the sheath while an assistant immobilizes the Y-connector on the guide catheter. This is a complex maneuver which should be practiced with a demonstration system before attempting it in a clinical situation. If not executed properly, the stent-delivery catheter will move with respect to its target site during the maneuver. The sheath should be retracted as far as the system allows (approximately 5 cm). The successful withdrawal of the sheath is confirmed by observing that the sheath marker has moved proximally with respect to the balloon-catheter markers (Fig. 4).

Once the sheath has been retracted, the exact location of the stent with respect to the lesion should be determined by angiography (Fig. 5). Care must be taken in interpreting the position of the stent because the force of the contrast-agent injection itself will frequently move the stent-delivery system several millimeters. It is essential to make sure that the Tuohy-Borst connector on the guide catheter is very tight in order to minimize the effects of the injection on the stent's position. It is undesirable (although feasible) to reposition the stent-delivery catheter once the stent is exposed. If the stent has been left proximal to the target site, it may snag on the vessel wall during attempts to advance it into position. If this occurs, there is no choice but to deploy the stent in an inappropriately proximal location. If the stent has been left distal to the target site, attempts to withdraw it into the correct position may cause it to slip off the balloon catheter, leaving it free and unexpanded in the lumen of the coronary artery. If an exposed unexpanded stent must be repositioned, careful attention must be paid to its location on the delivery catheter while moving it. This is not easily facilitated because of the stent's minimal radiopacity. If the stent begins to slip off the balloon, it should be expanded immediately to deploy it at its current location rather than attempt to move it farther.

Once the stent is exposed and the correct position within the target site has been verified by a contrast-agent injection and its relationship to landmarks, the balloon is prepared by applying vacuum for 30 seconds. A convenient preparation technique involves attaching the inflation device to the inflation port of the stent-delivery catheter with a three-way stopcock, and placing an empty 60-mL syringe on the sideport of the stopcock. The 60-mL syringe may be used to apply an intense vacuum to evacuate the air from the dead space of the balloon. Following this, the stopcock may be switched to connect the inflation-device syringe to the balloon-inflation lumen, and the balloon may be inflated in the conventional manner. The stent is deployed by inflating the balloon to a maximum inflation pressure of 6 ATM (rated burst pressure). The stent-delivery balloon customarily expands at the distal ends first and, subsequently, at the center as pressure is raised (Fig. 6). The distal ends of the stent offer the least resistance to expansion, and this property assists in anchoring the stent to the vascular wall. It is undesirable to rupture a balloon within a stent because of the possibility that the torn edge of the balloon might snag on the exposed tip of a stent strut, potentially precluding balloon withdrawal. Thus, one should not endeavor to achieve the definitive expansion of the stent with the stent-delivery balloon. After deployment, the stent-delivery balloon is deflated and the entire stent-delivery system is withdrawn completely from the guide catheter. The guidewire is left in position across the stent, and angiography is performed to assess the result (Fig. 7).

In general, further expansion of the stent is usually required to achieve the goal of a zero-residual stenosis or better. A conventional angioplasty balloon is introduced over the same guidewire, positioned within the stent, and inflated to further expand the stent and to achieve as large a lumen of the stented segment as possible (Fig. 8). The ideal balloon for this purpose is 15 mm in length (so that it does not impact on unstented segments of vessel), very strong (so that it can be inflated to 13- to 17-ATM pressure), and approximately 0.25 to 0.5 mm larger than the adjacent undiseased vessel. During this maneuver, it is important not to withdraw the tip of the guidewire into or proximal to the stent. If this occurs, it is possible that when the wire is readvanced, it may

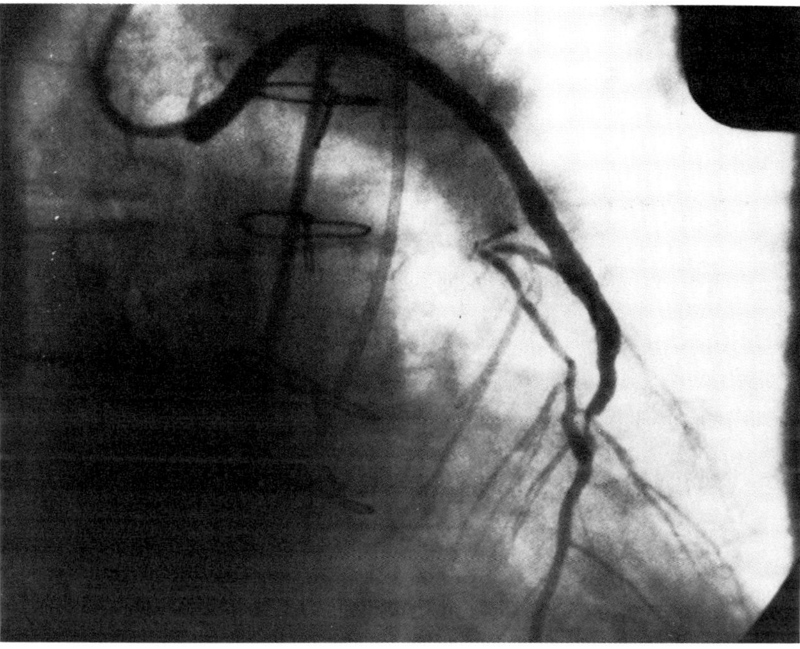

Figure 2: *A baseline angiogram showing a stenosis in a saphenous vein bypass graft just proximal to the anastomosis of the graft to the left anterior descending artery. Note that in this situation, placing the stent excessively distal would place it across the anastomosis.*

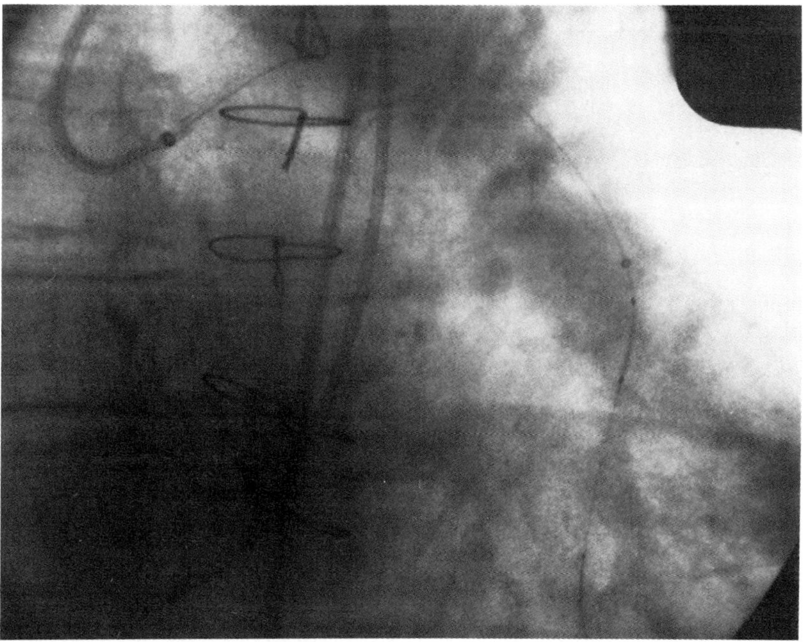

Figure 3: *The stent-delivery system in position in the region of the lesion. Note the position of the large marker on the sheath and the two smaller markers on the stent-delivery balloon. This is the relationship when the sheath is not retracted. Note also that the stent can be seen as a slight increase in radiographic density between the two markers on the balloon.*

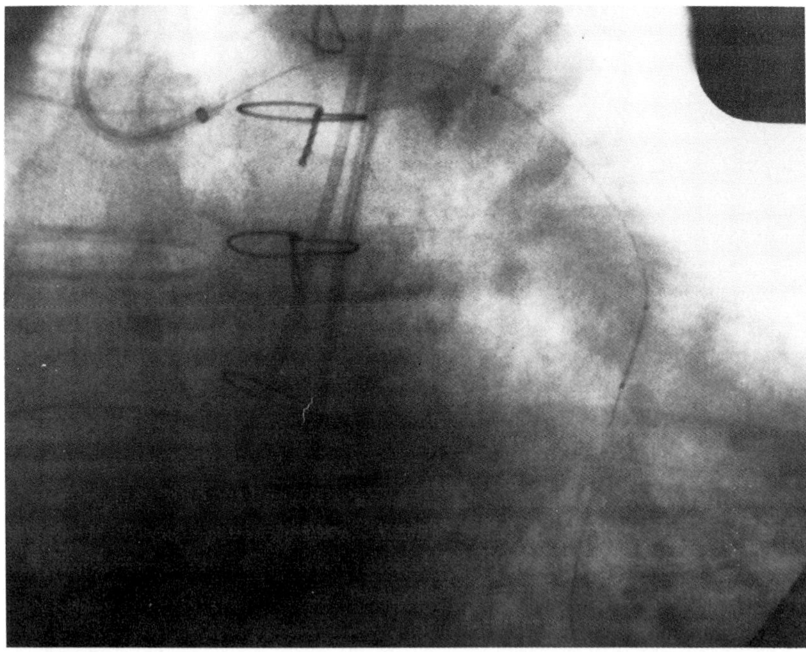

Figure 4: *The stent-delivery system in position in the region of the lesion, with the sheath retracted to expose the stent. Note that the marker on the sheath is now located more proximally along the catheter shaft.*

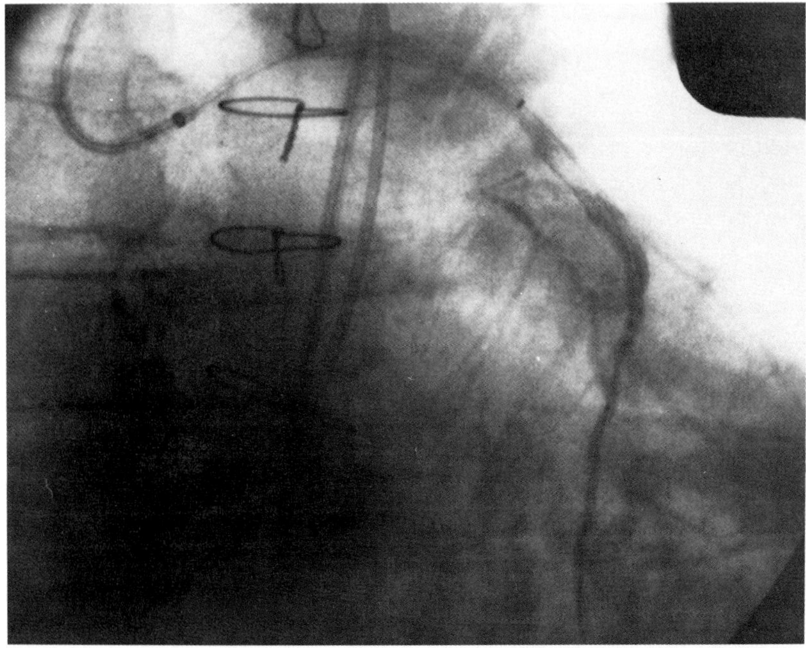

Figure 5: *An angiogram of the stent-delivery system in position, with the sheath retracted to assess the position of the stent. Note that filling of the vessel is poor because of the difficulty injecting contrast agent and obstruction of the vessel by the stent-delivery system. This angiogram discloses that the stent is approximately 3 mm too far, and needs to be repositioned before deployment.*

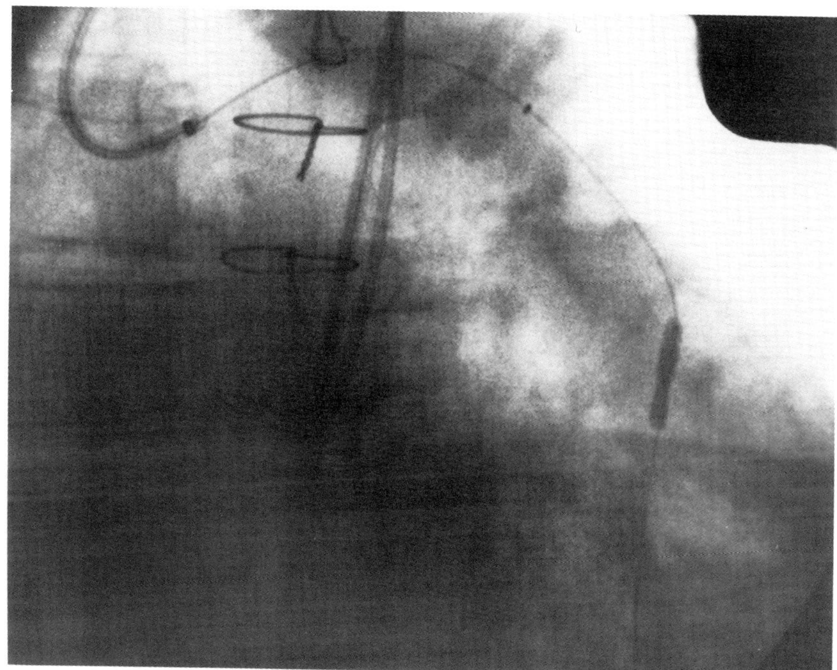

Figure 6: *Balloon inflation to deploy the stent. Note that the balloon inflates preferentially at its two ends.*

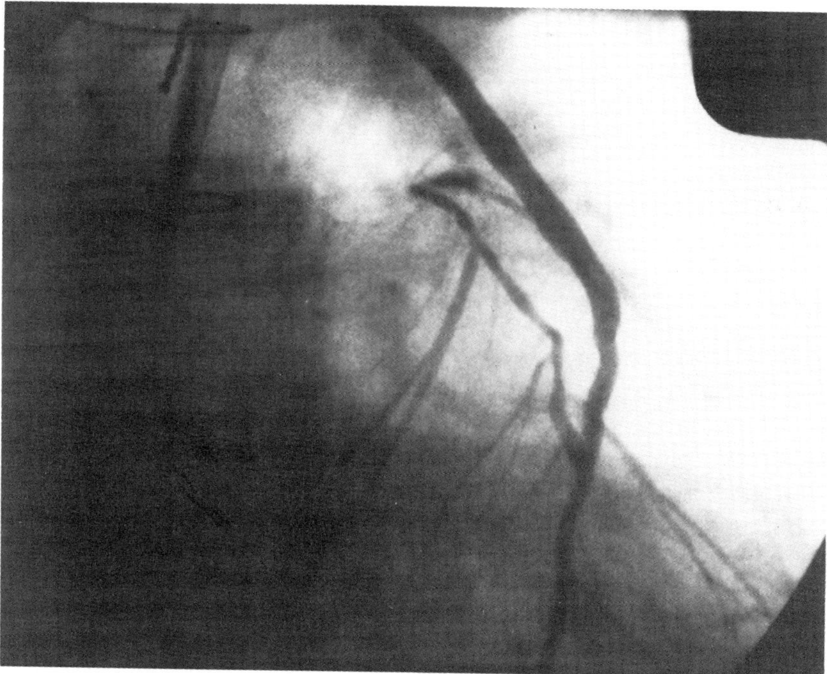

Figure 7: *The angiographic appearance of the vessel immediately following stent deployment with the stent-delivery balloon inflated to its maximum rated burst pressure of 6 ATM. Note the improvement in lumen dimension.*

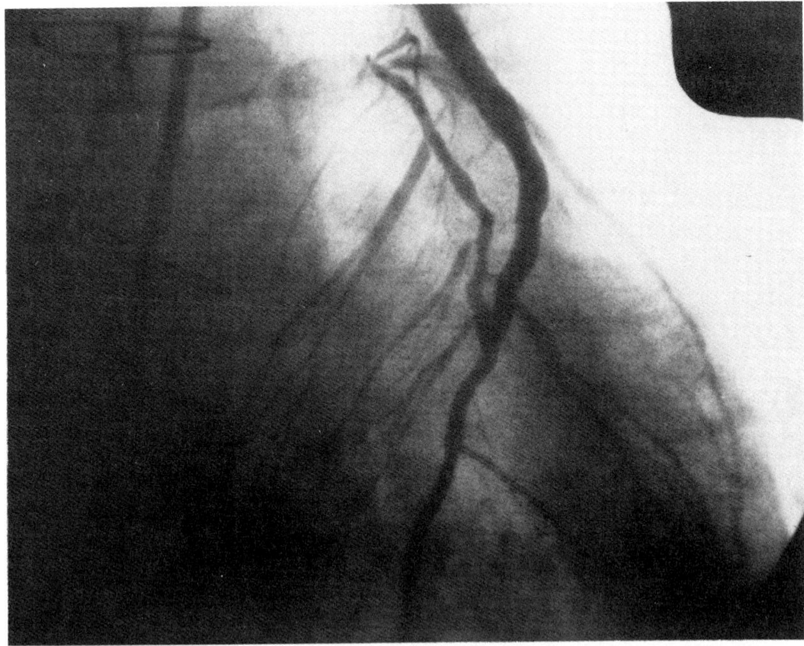

Figure 8: *The angiographic appearance of the vessel following further expansion of the stent with a 3.5-mm balloon. Note that the stent site is smooth with no irregularities, and that the diameter of the stented segment is matched to the diameter of the adjacent unstented vessel.*

pass between some of the stent struts and the vessel wall rather than cleanly through the lumen. It is almost impossible to recognize this phenomenon on fluoroscopy. If it does happen, attempts to advance another balloon catheter through the stent will bend portions of the stent away from the vascular wall, undermining the quality of the result and potentially making the site more thrombogenic. If resistance is encountered when attempting to advance another balloon catheter into position, this problem should be suspected and attempts to recross the stented segment should be abandoned. The Magnum wire (Schneider, Zurich, Switzerland), which has a 1-mm olive-shaped tip, may be useful in this situation because its blunt tip minimizes the likelihood of passing between the stent and the vessel wall.

Following the final overexpansion of the stent, the stented segment should be smooth and uniform (Fig. 8). There should be no irregularities within the lumen of the stent, and there should be no stenosis or dissection flap either immediately proximal or distal to the stent. Less than perfect results are at greater risk for later thrombosis[7] (see Chapter 8). The standards for what is an acceptable result of stenting are substantially higher than for conventional angioplasty. If further expansion is needed, there should be no hesitation to perform it. If there are unsealed dissection flaps or significant residual stenoses proximal or distal to the stent, serious consideration should be given to treating those areas with an additional stent.

Following final overexpansion of the stented segment, the patient should be observed for at least 10 minutes in the laboratory without withdrawing the guidewire. Repeat angiography should be performed at this point, with the guidewire in place. Of particular concern at this point is the possibility of early formation of thrombi within the stented segment. These appear as small lucencies or filling defects within the stented segment. A thrombus which accumulates early is an important predictor of later thrombosis and should be treated aggressively.[8] Appropriate strategies include redilation, which can mechanically disrupt the thrombus, and selective intracoronary infusion of thrombolytic agents. In extreme cases, prolonged selective infusion of thrombolytic agents has been used.

Other Considerations and Pitfalls of Stenting

General Considerations

Emergent Deployment

A number of emergent deployment situations arises in the practice of routine angioplasty. The most common circumstance indicating the use of a stent is an angioplasty-induced coronary dissection. If stenting is to be a viable alternative in this circumstance, it is important to be readily prepared to place the stent. Ideally, the guide catheter and guidewire that are already in place should be compatible with the stent-delivery system. If 7-F guides are used, replacement of the introducer sheath and the guide will be necessary in order to deliver a stent. If a .016-inch or .018-inch guidewire is used it will also need to be replaced. Finally, low-molecular weight dextran should be available in the laboratory so that it may be started immediately.

Position of the Stent on the Balloon Catheter

When the stent is crimped onto the balloon at the factory it is centered between the two markers. However, once it has been exposed, it may move either proximally or distally. This has major implications for deployment and for the possibility that the stent may slip off the balloon. Although the stent is not particularly radiopaque, it can be seen. Operators should train themselves to notice its location and use angiographic projections that offer the best visibility so that if the stent moves they can react appropriately.

Patient-Specific Considerations

Suitability for Warfarin Anticoagulation

When considering a patient for stenting, it is important to evaluate the patient as a candidate for the obligatory warfarin anticoagulation that must follow the implant. Because the patient must be treated with aspirin as well, the constraints on suitability for anticoagulation are more stringent.

Requirement for Surgery

If the patient requires any sort of surgical procedure during the anticoagulation period, a complex situation arises concerning anticoagulation management. The optimal strategy is to reverse the anticoagulation as little as possible for as short a period of time as is consistent with the demands of the surgical procedure. Obviously, an attempt to defer surgery during the first month should be made.

Proximal Vessel Considerations

Bends

Bends in proximal vessels which pose little difficulty for a conventional angioplasty catheter can be major obstacles for the stent-delivery system. The more severe the bend(s), the greater the requirement for guide-catheter support. The prototypical difficult situation is the "shepherd's crook" proximal right coronary artery. One of the more useful guide-catheter curves in this setting is the "hockey stick." Proper alignment of the tip of the guide catheter with the proximal coronary orifice and excellent bracing of the guide are both essential to achieve successful stent delivery.

Visualization of the Target Site

It is essential to determine the location of the target site accurately and to determine if the stent is properly positioned prior to deployment. In order to do this, it is necessary to have a radiological view which accurately displays the lesion and to be able to deliver an adequate amount of contrast agent to the deployment site. Larger lumen-guide catheters may be useful for vessels which have large proximal branches in order to deliver the contrast agent and accurately localize the target site.

Distance from the Orifice to the Target Site

The current stent-delivery system provides approximately 15 to 20 cm of useable length. Lesions which are fairly far down saphenous vein grafts, internal mammary arteries, or distal lesions in large right coronary arteries may not be reachable with the current version of the system.

Lesion Considerations

Preexisting Thrombus

The stent is a prothrombotic device. If it is inserted into a site that already has a thrombus attached to it, it will compound the propensity for thrombosis. This circumstance frequently occurs when considering the possibility of emergent deployment for failed angioplasty. It is important to attempt to determine whether the failure is due to dissection or a thrombus. Similarly, one should be careful not to use stents in angioplasty performed for acute myocardial infarction.

Poor Distal Runoff

Outflow of blood from the stented site is important to resist thrombosis and maintain patency. Therefore, stents should not be placed in a location that does not have good distal runoff.

Extremely Large Vessels

Extremely large vessels pose a problem because it may be difficult to achieve uniform contact of the stent with the vascular wall. A related problem is the vessel which has an aneurysmal segment immediately adjacent to the stent-deployment site, but which may be included within the stented segment. Such situations may be at greater risk of later thrombosis.

Deployment Considerations

Premature Sheath Withdrawal

If the sheath is withdrawn before the stent has reached the deployment position, it may not be possible to reach the target site, and one will be confronted with an exposed stent which cannot be delivered to the target site. There is little choice at this point other than to deploy the stent where it is in order not to risk embolizing it. A corollary of this situation is if the stent-delivery system cannot be advanced to the target site, one should never attempt to reach the target site by advancing the stent-delivery catheter past the tip of the sheath. This almost never works, and causes the above described problem.

Advancing the Sheath Past the End of the Balloon Catheter

The stent-delivery system is advanced by pushing on the sheath. If the sheath's Y-connector is not tightly locked to the stent-delivery catheter, the sheath can be pushed over the tip of the delivery catheter. It is important to be vigilant for this phenomenon by always observing the relationship between the marker on the sheath and the markers on the balloon.

Positioning for Very Short Lesions

If a lesion is very short, centering the stent on it may cause the lesion to fall within the articulation gap. In this circumstance, the stent should be placed either slightly more proximally or slightly more distally so that the lesion is supported by one of the two stent segments.

Positioning for Multiple Stents

If multiple stents (either tandem or not) are to be deployed in close proximity to each other, the plan for location of each relative to the others must be worked out prior to the deployment of the first stent. Otherwise, the location of earlier deployed stents may adversely affect the location of subsequently delivered stents.

REFERENCES

1. Schatz RA, Baim DS, Leon M, Ellis SG, Goldberg S, Hirshfeld JW, Cleman MW, Cabin HS, Walker C, Stagg J, Buchbinder M, Tierstein P, Topol EJ, Savage M, Perez JA, Curry RC, Whitworth H, Sousa JE, Tio FO, Almagor Y, Ponder LR, Penn IM, Leonard B, Levine SL, Fish DC, Palmaz JC: Clinical experience with the Palmaz-Schatz coronary stent: initial results of a multicenter study. *Circulation* 1991; 83: 148–161.
2. Baim DS, Bailey S, Curry C, Walker C, Schatz RA: Improved success and safety of Palmaz-Schatz coronary stenting with a new delivery system. *Circulation* 1990; 82(suppl III):III-657. Abstract.
3. Fishman DL, Savage MP, Leon MS, Schatz RA, Ellis S, Cleman MW, Hirshfeld JW Jr, Tierstein P, Bailey S, Walker CM, Goldberg S: Fate of lesion-related side branches following coronary artery stenting. *J Am Coll Cardiol* 1993 (in press).
4. Schatz RA: A view of vascular stents. *Circulation* 1989; 79:445–457.
5. Ellis SG, Savage M, Fischman D, Baim DS, Leon M, Goldberg S, Hirshfeld JW, Cleman MW, Tierstein PS, Walker C, Bailey S, Buchbinder M, Topol EJ, Schatz RA: Restenosis after placement of Palmaz-Schatz stents in native coronary arteries: initial results of a multicenter experience. *Circulation* 1992; 86:1836–1844.
6. Macaya C, Alfonso F, Iniguez A, Goicolea J, Hernandez R, Zarco P: Stenting for elastic recoil during coronary angioplasty of the left main coronary artery. *Am J Cardiol* 1992; 70:105–107.
7. Fischman DL, Savage MP, Leon MB, Hirshfeld JW, Cleman MW, Tierstein P, Goldberg S: Angiographic predictors of subacute thrombosis following coronary artery stenting. *Circulation* 1991; 84(suppl II):II-558.
8. Herrmann HC, Buchbinder M, Cleman MW, Fischman D, Goldberg S, Leon MB, Schatz RA, Tierstein P, Walker CM, Hirshfeld JW: Emergent use of balloon expandable coronary artery stenting for failed PTCA. *Circulation* 1992; 86:812–819.

CHAPTER 3

Antithrombotic Therapy Before and After Stent Deployment

Elliot S. Barnathan

The vessel wall normally provides a nonthrombogenic surface which helps contribute to blood fluidity. There are several important broad areas in which the vessel wall participates in maintaining this state that can be categorized as: 1) antiplatelet mechanisms, 2) anticoagulant mechanisms, and 3) profibrinolytic mechanisms. Endothelial cells, which line the luminal surface are normally nonadherent for platelets, and secrete antiplatelet substances such as prostacyclin (PGI_2) which help to inhibit platelet activation near the vessel wall. In addition, they can express receptor molecules on their surface, such as thrombomodulin, which promote the generation of anticoagulant factors. The endothelium also releases profibrinolytic compounds such as tissue-type (t-PA) and urokinase-type plasminogen activator (u-PA) which can bind to endothelial cell receptors and increase the local generation of plasmin.

Although the unperturbed endothelium has evolved to possess many antithrombotic mechanisms, it was equally important evolutionarily, for the endothelium to be able to promptly respond to vascular injury by becoming procoagulant. The mammalian vasculature has developed the capacity to rapidly: 1) become stimulatory toward platelets enabling platelet adhesion and aggregation; 2) generate tissue factor and other procoagulant proteins; 3) express normally cryptic-binding sites for coagulation factors which accelerate coagulant reactions; and 4) increase the expression of antifibrinolytic compounds such as plasminogen activator inhibitor type 1 (for review see[1]). However, few vascular injuries encountered in evolution lead to rapid near complete loss of the endothelium such as that which occurs after balloon angioplasty. Rapid platelet deposition occurs with subsequent platelet aggregation and release causing further platelet recruitment, the generation of thrombin which further activates platelets and generates fibrin which together may lead to thrombosis.

From: Herrmann HC, Hirshfeld JW, eds. *Clinical Use of the Palmaz-Schatz Intracoronary Stent.* Futura Publishing Company, Inc., Mount Kisco, NY, © 1993.

Heparin alone has been demonstrated to be inadequate to inhibit thrombosis after angioplasty.[2] Several studies have now demonstrated the efficacy of antiplatelet agents such as aspirin,[2,3] ticlopidine,[4] prostacyclin or more stable analogs such as ciprostene in reducing acute complications after percutaneous transluminal coronary angioplasty (PTCA).[5] Standard current therapy with aspirin and intravenous heparin has reduced the acute closure rate to ~2% to 7%,[6–8] except in patients with preexistent thrombus who continue to have a higher acute complication rate[9] unless pretreated with heparin.[10]

The advent of intracoronary stent deployment has added yet an additional challenge to the cardiologist in terms of still new mechanisms of thrombogenesis which may require even more potent therapy. All foreign surfaces developed to date, to a greater or lesser extent, are adherent for platelets and may stimulate aggregation. In addition, many foreign surfaces, particularly negatively charged ones as well as proteoglycan containing subendothelial matrix exposed in the vessel wall after conventional balloon angioplasty, may activate and/or bind contact factors such as factor XII and high-molecular weight kininogen, ultimately leading to factor Xa generation which mediates factor V activation, generating thrombin and, ultimately, fibrin. Rheologic factors may work in favor or against thrombosis after stent deployment depending on the degree of expansion of the stent, and the underlying lesion composition. Prior to stent deployment, the presence of angiographically-visible thrombus has been suggested as a strong predictor of total occlusion, presumably via a thrombotic mechanism.[11] In fact, to date, the major Achilles heel of stent deployment has been the problem of subacute thrombosis within the first week. Considering all of the natural antiplatelet, anticoagulant, and fibrinolytic mechanisms that may be compromised by both angioplasty and/or stent deployment, the successful use of the current generation of stents requires careful attention to the design of a potent but safe antithrombotic regimen. Alterations in the biocompatibility and thromboresistance properties of the stents themselves may aid in this process, although no truly thromboresistant surface has been generated to date.

Principles of Antithrombotic Therapy

The major focus of antithrombotic therapy for the patient receiving an intracoronary stent is to prevent platelet activation and intravascular coagulation. Therefore, it is important to understand some basic aspects of platelet physiology and the coagulation system (Fig. 1).

Platelets

Platelet activation is usually considered to consist of four processes: 1) adhesion (usually to exposed subendothelial matrix components such as collagen; 2) shape change (from normal discoid to an irregular shape with pseudo-

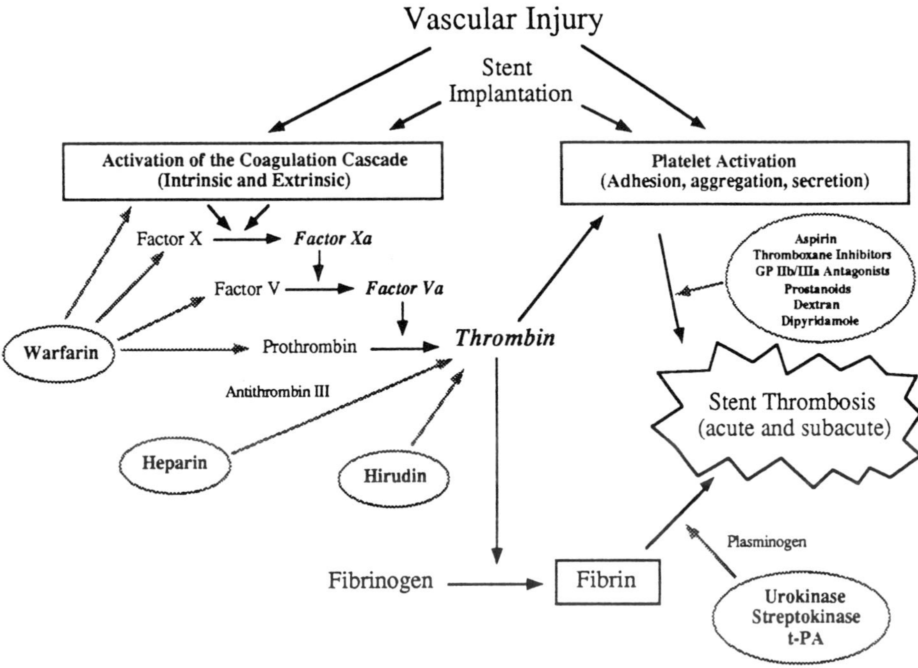

Figure 1: *Interactions of the coagulation cascade and platelet activation leading to stent thrombosis.*

podia); 3) secretion (of granular contents); and 4) aggregation. There are many substances which have been demonstrated to activate platelets via a variety of different pathways, such as thrombin, epinephrine, and thromboxane A_2 (which all bind to specific cell surface receptors) and initiate a cascade of signal-transducing reactions leading to platelet activation. Antiplatelet agents may prevent activation by some pathways, but not others. Aspirin irreversibly inactivates cyclo-oxygenase in platelets, thus rendering them incapable of generating thromboxane A_2 when stimulated. However, aspirinated-platelets can still aggregate to thrombin, which is undoubtedly generated in or around the implanted stent. Other novel agents, such as monoclonal antibodies to the glycoprotein IIb/IIIa, prevent aggregation from multiple stimuli, since their mechanism of action is to prevent fibrinogen-dependent bridging between platelets, regardless of the mode of stimulation. It is expected that agents such as this will be rather potent, causing a globally decreased platelet responsiveness, and will have a long duration of action. Since there will be little chance for reversal of this effect acutely, titrating the degree of platelet inhibition in the setting of a recent intravascular procedure may be difficult. Prostanoid agents, such as prostacyclin or its analogs (e.g., iloprost, ciprostene), are potent antiplatelet agents even when challenged with very large artificial surfaces, such as during extracorporeal circulation. Since these agents have a very short half-life, they can be turned off after the extracorporeal circulation is finished, with a rapid return of normal platelet function. Due to preservation of platelets in an intact fashion, less bleeding has actually been observed clinically with their use during open heart surgery. Iloprost has been shown to prevent platelet activation in a superior fashion to aspirin during bypass surgery in patients with heparin-associated thrombocytopenia who must receive heparin.[12] Ciprostene has been demonstrated to be effective in preventing acute complications when used during conventional PTCA,[5], although no trial to date has evaluated the efficacy of a prostanoid after stent deployment.

Coagulation Factors

Although platelets are the first line of defense against hemorrhage, cross-linked fibrin needs to be generated to stabilize and strengthen the platelet aggregate and form the mature thrombus. Activated platelets form an initial plug to stop bleeding and also provide a catalytic surface for the assembly and interaction of coagulation factors. Factors V and VIII interact and, subsequently, activate factors X and II to form the prothrombinase complex. This complex ultimately generates thrombin which acts on fibrinogen to make fibrin-I monomers. After polymerization of fibrin-I monomers, thrombin can cleave this polymer, resulting in fibrin II generation. Thrombin can also activate factor XI and thus positively feed back via the intrinsic pathway which eventually leads to factor IXa-VIIa-mediated generation of factor Xa on cell surfaces. The second classical pathway, which is the primary one in vivo for the activation of factor X, is termed the extrinsic pathway which uses tissue factor bound to factor VIIa for factor Xa generation. Recent work has also demonstrated that tissue factor-VIIa complex can activate factor IX as well.

Two major mechanisms for controlling these pathways involve the interaction of circulating factors with the components of the vascular wall. Antithrombin III can bind to thrombin, factor XIa, and factor Xa, with this reaction being greatly enhanced by either exogenously added heparin, or by endogenous heparinlike substances associated with the endothelium such as heparan sulfate. Even in the presence of heparin, antithrombin III is a poor inhibitor of clot-bound thrombin,[13] which has stimulated the recent interest in developing novel thrombin inhibitors, such as hirudin, which will inactivate thrombin bound to the clot. In a baboon endovascular stent model, heparin was ineffective at preventing thrombus formation, while D-FPRDH_2Cl, a synthetic antithrombin, blocked thrombus formation.[14] Antistasin is a naturally occurring factor Xa inhibitor which is under development as a novel anticoagulant. Thrombin can also bind to thrombomodulin, a protein found on the endothelial cell surface. After binding, thrombin can mediate the activation of circulating protein C. Activated protein C can, in turn, in the presence of a cofactor called protein S, inhibit the coagulation cascade at several points including inhibition of factors Va and VIIIa.[15] An additional inhibitory protein has recently been identified, known either as lipoprotein-associated coagulation inhibitor (LACI) or the extrinsic pathway inhibitor (EPI). This protein inhibits factor VIIa-dependent activation of factor Xa.[16] The loss of endothelium and its thrombomodulin after PTCA and stent deployment could thereby remove normal anticoagulant mechanisms. Studies using recombinant protein inhibitors of the coagulation pathway in association with stent deployment have not been reported.

Oral anticoagulants have now been shown by several groups[17–19] to be mandatory adjunctive pharmacologic agents in the patient receiving an intracoronary stent. Warfarin sodium, and other drugs in its class, act by antagonizing the actions of vitamin K and inhibiting the synthesis of several blood clotting proteins including prothrombin, factor VII, factor IX and factor X.[20] Vitamin K antagonism also inhibits important posttranslation modifications of protein C and protein S. After initiation of anticoagulation therapy with warfarin, the circulating levels of these factors begin to decrease based on their half-lives. Levels of factor VII, (half-life = ~ 6 hours), are found to be rapidly depressed, whereas levels of prothrombin (half-life = ~ 72 hours) drop off much more slowly. Since the measured prothrombin time (PT) is highly dependent on the factor VII level, one may have a situation 2 to 4 days after the start of warfarin therapy, where the PT is prolonged, yet levels of other factors are not substantially suppressed. For that reason, many researchers have suggested overlapping heparin therapy for some period of time to ensure adequate suppression of factor levels before discontinuing the heparin. Similarly, the depression of protein C and protein S levels can be procoagulant and the maintenance of heparin therapy for an extended period during the initiation of warfarin therapy may mitigate these negative effects. The timing of many subacute occlusions poststenting would argue for inadequate oral anticoagulation as a significant contributing factor.

Work by Other Investigators

Table 1 outlines the antithrombotic regimens used by representative groups of investigators with three of the intracoronary stents that have had the widest testing to date in the published literature. A review of the literature has demonstrated that, in virtually all series,[17- 19,21,22] an evolution of antithrombotic strategies has occurred, usually with an increasing intensity of antithrombotic therapy due to a higher than acceptable percentage of early failures. Nevertheless, this has not been without additional risk, in that there has been an increased number of groin complications, principally hematomas and pseudoaneurysms, some requiring surgery.

It has been clear from the initial report of stent deployment in humans[21] that acute or subacute closure, presumably by thrombus, was a problem. Sigwart noted two documented occlusions out of 19 patients with a third, not documented, resulting in death. In a later review of data from the Wallstent investigators, Serruys noted 21 subacute occlusions 1 to 14 days after implantation, with 25 occlusions in the entire series (24%). It was noted that 39% of the patients with occlusion were at one center which initially did not use oral

Table 1.
Acute and Chronic Therapy

Acute Therapy
(Prestent, Peristent)

Type of Stent	*ASA*	*Dipyridamole*	*Heparin*	*Thrombolytic*	*Calcium Blocker*	*NTG*	*Dextran*
Palmaz-Schatz	325mg qD 24-48 h pre	75 mg TID 24–48 h pre	10,000 U bolus, 2500 U/hr ACT 2–2.5 baseline	Only if thrombus visible pre or post stent ≤500,000 U	yes 24 h pre	200 μg IC pre and post stent	LMW Dextran (Dextran 40), start 2 h pre at 50–100 ml/h until 1 liter infused.
Gianturco-Roubin	325 mg × 2 doses	yes (? dose)	10,000 U bolus additional as needed ACT >300 sec	Some pts 80,000 U/h urokinase for 12–18 h	?	100–200 μg IC	Only pt thought at high risk (Dextran 40, 10%, at 50–75 ml/h for at least 2 h pre; 100 ml–200 ml Dextran 40 bolus at time of stent; then 100 ml/h × 2 h, then 50 ml/hr until sheaths pulled.)
Wallstent	1 g 1 d pre	300 mg qD 1 d pre	10–15,000 bolus with SQ hepartin TID started 3d pre to maintain ACT 2 × control	100,000 U urokinase IC	?	?	?

Chronic Therapy *Poststent*

Type of Stent	ASA	Dipyridamole	Oral anticoagulant	Calcium Blocker	Acute Occlusion*	Subacute Occlusion	All occlusions*	Reference
Palmaz-Schatz	yes × 3 m	yes × 3 m	warfarin × 3 m	yes × 3 m	0/226 (0%)	8/226 (3.5%)	8/228 (3.5%)	Schatz[17]
Gianturco-Roubin	yes, indefinitely	yes × 2 m	warfarin × 2 m	?	7/108 (6.5%)	7/108 (6.5%)	14/108 (13%)	Roubin[18]
Wallstent	1g initially then 100 mg qD	300–450 mg qD	acenocoumarol × 3–6 m (in later patients)	?	N/A	21/105 (23.8%)	25/105 (23.8%)	Serruys[19]

* Indications for stenting varied between these series and therefore occlusion rates cannot be directly compared.

Table 2.
Predictors of Subacute Thrombosis Following Intracoronary Stenting

	Reference
Inadequate anticoagulation	26, 19, 17
Intraprocedural thrombus before or after stent	23, 26, 27
Residual stenosis higher	23
Dissection present poststent	23
Residual intimal dissection	23
Eccentricity	26
Residual distal vessel irregularity poststent	44
Bailout indication	44, 27
Unstable angina	44
Type-C lesion	44
Lesion length > 1.5 cm	44
Plaque area > 3.5 cm^2	44
Symptomatic post-PTCA dissection	44
Incomplete wrapping of dissection	44

anticoagulation and used a low dose of aspirin (100 mg, 1 day prior to stenting). These investigators now use heparin subcutaneously for 3 days prior to implantation and routinely administer low doses of intracoronary urokinase (100,000 IU).[19] Most other investigators have not used thrombolytic agents routinely unless flow was compromised or intrastent thrombus was documented.

Fischman and coworkers[11] studied predictors of subacute thrombosis and identified higher residual stenosis, dissection present after stenting, and thrombus present before or after stenting as significant risk factors (see Chapter 8). Haude et al also noted several predictors of subacute thrombosis (see Table 2). The strongest predictor was residual distal vessel irregularity present after stenting. Overall, the rates for subacute stent thrombosis have ranged from 0% to 30%, depending on the type of lesion stented and the antithrombotic regimen used. Schatz[17] noted an 18% (7/39) incidence of subacute occlusion in the absence of chronic oral anticoagulation, but only one in 174 subsequent patients receiving warfarin developed subacute occlusion. Despite this very promising initial result, all of these patients were elective, prospectively enrolled patients with coronary artery disease, without acute myocardial infarction or abrupt closure after PTCA. In the largest series of Palmaz-Schatz stent implantations to date,[23] the overall subacute thrombosis rate was 5.2% (38/726). Fischman reported a higher incidence of subacute thrombosis when the original indication for implantation was impending occlusion rather than for restenosis.[23]

Sutton reviewed data from 392 patients receiving the Gianturco-Roubin stent for acute closure and compared it to data from 205 patients receiving the same stent for restenosis. Patients receiving a stent for acute closure had a higher rate of subacute closure (9.4% versus 3.4%), acute closure (8.2% versus 1.0%), and bypass surgery, infarction, and death (20.7% versus 9.8%).[24] A similar high-subacute occlusion rate has been noted with the Strecker stent (10/51 or 19.6%) when used for acute occlusion post-PTCA.[25] Nath[26] reported on a series of 145 patients receiving a stent for abrupt closure or restenosis. Of the 17 patients with any occlusion, (7 acute $<$ 24 hours),10 subacute $>$ 24 hours), all had at least one partial thromboplastin time (PTT) documented at less than twice control or a PT less then 1.4x control, compared to 20/33 stent patients without occlusion. In only two out of 17 patients was the value low due to bleeding, prompting the decreased strength of anticoagulation whereas in 11 of 33 patients without occlusion this was the case. These investigators have noted again that the presence of thrombus or eccentric stenoses predisposed to occlusion. Herrmann et al have examined a particularly high-risk group of patients who all received stents as an emergency.[27] The subacute closure rate was 16.6% (9/54) with myocardial infarction (MI), coronary artery bypass graft (CABG), or death in 27.8% (15/54). The subgroup with acute closure rather than impending closure or suboptimal results after PTCA seemed to be at the highest risk. Of note, there were eight major groin complications, mainly pseudoaneurysms, and seven nongroin hemorrhagic complications.

A potential mechanism for avoiding acute occlusions or identifying the patients most at risk so as to minimize the need for higher strength anticoagulation, would be to identify more accurate laboratory tests to detect subclinical thrombosis before it becomes occlusive. Erbel et al have used monitoring of fragment $_{1.2}$ which is generated in vivo when prothrombin is activated, and has been advocated as a sensitive marker of ongoing thrombosis.[28] In a series of 54 patients monitored and treated conventionally, subacute thrombosis was noted in nine (17%). After instituting monitoring of fragment $_{1.2}$ and readjusting the strength of anticoagulation based on it, subacute thrombosis has only occurred once in 32 patients (3.1%). Further validation of this promising strategy seems warranted.

Recommendations for Antithrombotic Therapy: Prestent Management

With the realizations that antithrombotic therapy for stent patient is both critically important and potentially dangerous, and that, at best, it involves a large degree of empiricism in the absence of firm clinical research data, we propose the following recommendations and guidelines for therapy. These are based on the collective experiences of the stent investigators outlined above, and upon basic principles of antithrombotic therapy.

Antiplatelet Therapy

Some form of antiplatelet therapy is mandatory. Aspirin should be given (not enteric-coated) in a dose of at least 324 mg, at least 30 to 60 minutes prior to PTCA , preferably starting therapy the day prior to the procedure. Several doses will ensure adequate efficacy, particularly if bioavailability is variable as it can be with enteric-coated preparations, which should be avoided for that reason. If stent deployment is an emergency, aspirin should be chewed for optimal bioavailability. Most investigators have continued to utilize dipyridamole in addition to aspirin.

Although some retrospective data suggested that chronic treatment with both aspirin and dipyridamole compared to aspirin alone was associated with a decreased amount of acute thrombus formation complicating routine PTCA,[2] this was not confirmed in a prospective randomized controlled trial.[29] Nevertheless, dipyridamole has been a safe and useful adjunct to chronic warfarin therapy in patients with artificial valves, where there are also issues of blood/artificial surface interaction. There are also vasodilatory properties of dipyridamole which could improve rheologic factors independently of its purported antiplatelet efficacy. In the absence of additional data to support withdrawal of dipyridamole from the standard regimen, we continue to support its use beginning 24 to 48 hours before stent implantation. Ticlopidine can be used in aspirin-allergic patients. This agent has been shown to be as efficacious as aspirin in inhibiting acute complications of routine PTCA.[4] Monitoring of complete blood counts every 2 weeks is mandatory during ticlopidine therapy because of rare, reversible, but potentially severe neutropenia.

Dextrans are plasma expanders which can inhibit platelet function in vivo as evidenced by prolonged bleeding times. Decreased platelet aggregation and impaired platelet procoagulant activity have also been reported.[30] Several different regimens have been used (see Table 1). Our recommendation is to use a dextran product (e.g., Dextran 40), starting 2 hours preprocedure at 50 to 100 ml per hour until one liter is infused. Some older studies suggested that the higher molecular weight products have a greater effect on hemostasis.[31]

Anticoagulation

As with routine PTCA procedures, adequate heparinization is important. There are no other substitutes currently available, although novel direct-thrombin inhibitors are currently being evaluated in clinical trials. An initial intravenous bolus of 10,000 to 15,000 U of heparin is normally followed by additional small doses to maintain the activated clotting time (ACT) above 300 seconds. Activated clotting time values below 250 have been associated with increased major complications during routine angioplasty,[32] and some investigators have suggested lower acute thrombotic complications of routine PTCA when the ACT was maintained above 350 or 400 seconds.

Fibrinolytic Therapy

No clear consensus has developed as to the utility of the routine use of fibrinolytic agents such as streptokinase, urokinase, or t-PA as adjuncts to routine PTCA or stent implantation. Despite its potent ability to lyse thrombi, fibrinolytic therapy has also been associated with increased thrombin activity,[33] possibly by exposing thrombin trapped inside the dissolving thrombus. Platelet activation has also been demonstrated after fibrinolytic therapy due perhaps, in part, to direct activation by plasmin, but more likely indirectly via plasmin-mediated activation of the coagulation system generating thrombin which subsequently activates platelets.[34] Streptokinase has also been demonstrated to cause platelet aggregation by binding antistreptokinase antibodies to streptokinase-plasminogen complexes on the platelet surface.[35] However, platelet inhibition or disaggregation has also been later documented after fibrinolytic therapy, possibly mediated by plasmin cleavage of platelet-related proteins.[36–38] Given the significant increased risk of bleeding including intracranial hemorrhage with fibrinolytic agents, their routine use cannot currently be advocated. However, some have suggested that the addition of agents such as urokinase during complicated angioplasty can be associated with a favorable outcome.[39] Whether fibrinolytic therapy administered to patients at high risk of acute or subacute thrombosis, such as those with angiographically-visible thrombus, will reduce the incidence of these negative outcomes remains to be determined. If flow is limiting despite successful stent deployment, intracoronary fibrinolytic agents have been successful in reestablishing flow and preventing at least a portion of these patients from requiring emergency CABG.

Poststent Management

The major problem in the immediate poststent period is how to decrease the level of anticoagulation enough to enable the safe removal of sheaths. One must strive to minimize the time period with a reduced intensity of anticoagulation, achieve adequate hemostasis, and quickly reestablish an adequate level of anticoagulation. Various strategies to accomplish this have been suggested, and must be adapted to the individual practitioner's settings. In general, it is preferable to discontinue the intravenous heparin infusion at a time when physicians are available to monitor coagulation parameters and patient symptoms. We have utilized the ACT because it is rapid, easy to perform, inexpensive, and gives a reasonable estimate of the degree of heparinization. Some have favored an ACT value of less than 150 seconds prior to sheath removal.[18] Once hemostasis is achieved, heparin should be restarted either immediately or within 4 hours, preferably with a small bolus, and a continuous I.V. infusion. Early monitering of the PTT is essential to ensure adequate anticoagulation with proper dosage adjustments, ultimately maintaining the levels at least twice the normal value. Antiplatelet therapy with aspirin is strongly recommended. No clear consensus has developed, but even low doses given chronically nearly completely block platelet-thromboxane A_2 synthesis. Most groups have also used dipyridamole as well, for 2 to 3 months.

The conversion to chronic anticoagulation with warfarin or its derivatives is now recognized as mandatory with most stents being tested. Because of the early increase in the measured PT despite inadequate suppression of certain coagulation factors with long half-lives, we extend the heparin anticoagulation for at least 24 hours beyond the time of stable, therapeutic PT elevation. The appropriate strength of anticoagulation is not clear. Most investigators at United States centers with the Palmaz-Schatz stent aim for a PT of 16 to 18 seconds,[17,23] while investigators using the Gianturco-Roubin stent aim for 17 to 20 seconds.[40] Other groups have reported target international normalized ratio (INRs) of greater than 2.3, [41] less than 2.5,[21,42] or even as high as 2.8 to 4.3.[43] In this last study using the Palmaz-Schatz stent exclusively for acute occlusion or dissection complicating PTCA, there were six subacute occlusions in 127 patients from 3 to 11 days after stent deployment (4.7%) despite this high level of anticoagulation, and 11 patients had "severe" bleeding complications.[43] Early results with fragment $F_{1.2}$ monitoring have been promising as a marker of ongoing thrombosis and the need for increased anticoagulation, but this needs to be validated in larger series.

The degree of anticoagulation must be carefully considered for each individual patient. Those patients with risk factors for subacute thrombosis should be more closely monitored and should perhaps have a longer period of overlap between heparin and warfarin with a higher level of anticoagulation. Thrombus visible angiographically before and/or after stent placement, residual intimal dissection, or residual distal vessel irregularity have been identified as strong predictors of subsequent stent occlusion.[23,27,44] Bailout indication, type-C lesion, lesion length greater than 1.5 cm, and plaque area greater than 3.5 cm^2 have also been suggested as significant risk factors.[44] Anticoagulation is routinely continued for 1 to 2 months. In most animal studies and in the limited data available from humans, it would appear that an intact endothelial lining has usually regrown in this time period, and may decrease the need for extended anticoagulation. This must, however, be individualized depending on the underlying nature of the lesion, the status of the artery after stenting, and the clinical condition of the patient. Long-term studies of anticoagulation versus no anticoagulation have not been performed to date, but may be necessitated as long-term follow-up data accumulates. Antiplatelet therapy should be continued indefinitely.

Future Directions

The current requirement for intensive antithrombotic therapy after stent placement has created much enthusiasm for modifying stents in such a way as to make them less thrombogenic, or to make them able to deliver drugs locally to prevent or dissolve local thrombus.

One novel approach has been to seed metallic stents with autologous endothelial cells in the hope of a faster reendothelialization to decrease both thrombosis and restenosis. Dichek and coworkers have demonstrated that this is technically feasible in sheep, with some retention of the endothelial cells on the external and lateral surfaces of the preseeded Palmaz-Schatz stent.[45] In this study, the autologous endothelial cells were able to be transfected ex vivo with either a reporter gene or with a potentially useful gene (for t-PA) in the hope of eventually secreting the protein locally in high concentration. Others have demonstrated direct gene transfer into the arterial wall[46,47] using catheter-based techniques which, in the future, could be combined with intracoronary stenting.

Several novel adjunctive pharmacologic therapies are already in various phases of clinical trials for various aspects of the treatment of ischemic heart disease. Some are currently being studied as adjuncts during routine PTCA, but it is likely that some will also be tried in the setting of intracoronary stenting. A partial list of the types of agents under investigation (and representative examples) include: 1) novel thrombin inhibitors, such as hirudin, hirulog, argatroban; 2) glycoprotein-IIb/IIIa antagonists, including monoclonal antibodies such as 7E3 and integrelin (a synthetic peptide antagonist); 3) prostacyclin and its analogs, such as betaprost, taprostene, ciprostene, eptaloprost, and iloprost; 4) thromboxane-A_2 antagonists, such as sulotroban and daltroban; 5) thromboxane-A_2 synthetase inhibitors, such as ozagrel, rolafagrel; 6) plasminogen activators such as prourokinase and r-PA; 7) heparin subfractions such as enoxaparin, logiparin, normiflow; and 8) heparinlike compounds such as tedelparin, mucoglucoronan, and naroparil.

An additional novel approach has been the concept of combining pharmacologic therapy with intracoronary stenting. Several bioabsorbable stents have been constructed out of different materials such as purified type-1 collagen.[48] Some of these stents have the capacity to have drugs added during their synthesis, and could function as a slow-release device as well. Others have begun to look at various coatings on stents such as heparin, which can be covalently bonded to the surface, or more biological coatings such as fibrin.[49] Over the next several years, the interdisciplinary collaborative efforts of bioengineers, biomaterials scientists, pharmacologists, biochemists, cellular and molecular biologists, hematologists, and cardiologists will hopefully lead to the development of less thrombogenic stents for human use or, at least, safer, more effective pharmacologic strategies for preventing complications with their use.

REFERENCES

1. Jaffe EA: Endothelial cell structure and function. In: Hoffman R, Benz EJ Jr, Shattil SJ, Furie B, Cohen HJ, eds. *Hematology: Basic Principles and Practice.* New York: Churchill Livingstone; 1991:1198.
2. Barnathan ES, Schwartz JS, Taylor L, Laskey WK, Kleaveland JP, Kussmaul WG, Hirshfeld JW Jr: Aspirin and dipyridamole in the prevention of acute coronary thrombosis complicating coronary angioplasty. *Circulation* 1987; 76:125.
3. Schwartz L, Bourassa MG, Lesperance J, Aldridge HE, Kazim F, Salvatori VA, Henderson M, Bonan R, David PR: Aspirin and dipyridamole in the prevention of restenosis after percutaneous transluminal coronary angioplasty. *New Eng J Med* 1988; 318:1714.
4. Bertrand ME, Allain H, Lablanche JM: Results of a randomized trial of ticlopidine

versus placebo for prevention of acute closure and restenosis after coronary angioplasty (PTCA): The TACT Study. *Circulation* 1990; 82(suppl III):III-190. Abstract.
5. Raizner A, Hollman J, Demke D, Wakefield L: Beneficial effects of ciprostene in PTCA: a multicenter, randomized, controlled trial. *Circulation* 1988; 78(suppl II): II-290. Abstract.
6. deFeyter PJ, van den Brand M, Jaarman G, van Domburg R, Serruys PW, Suryapranata H: Acute coronary artery occlusion during and after percutaneous transluminal coronary angioplasty. *Circulation* 1991; 83:927.
7. Stammen F, Peissens J, Vrolix M, Glazier JJ, De Geest H, Willems JL: Immediate and short-term results of a 1988–1989 coronary angioplasty registry. *Am J Cardiol* 1991; 67:253.
8. Detre KM, Holmes DR, Holubkov R, Cowley MJ, Bourassa MG, Faxon DP, Dorros GR, Bentivoglio LG, Kent KM, Myler RK: Incidence and consequences of periprocedural occlusion. *Circulation* 1990; 82:739.
9. Mabin TA, Holmes DR, Smith HC, Vliestra TE, Bove AA, Reeder GS, Chesebro JM, Bresnahan JF, Orszulak TA: Intracoronary thrombus: role in coronary occlusion complicating percutaneous transluminal coronary angioplasty. *J Am Coll Cardiol* 1985; 5:198.
10. Laskey MA, Deutsch E, Hirshfeld JW Jr, Kussmaul WG, Barnathan E, Laskey WK: Influence of heparin therapy on percutaneous transluminal coronary angioplasty outcome in patients with coronary arterial thrombus. *Am J Cardiol* 1990; 65:179.
11. Fischman DL, Savage MP, Leon MB, Schatz RA, Ellis SG, Cleman MW, Teirstein P, Walker CM, Bailey S, Hirshfeld JW, Goldberg S: Effect of intracoronary stenting on intimal dissection after balloon angioplasty: results of quantitative and qualitative coronary analysis. *J Am Coll Cardiol* 1991; 18:1445.
12. Kappa JR, Horn M III, Fisher CA, Cottrell ED, Ellison N, Addonizio VP: Efficacy of iloprost (ZK36374) versus aspirin in preventing heparin-induced platelet activation during cardiac operations. *J Thorac Cardiovasc Surg* 1987; 94:405.
13. Teitel JM, Rosenberg RD: Protection of factor Xa from neutralization by the heparin-antithrombin complex. *J Clin Invest* 1983; 71:1383.
14. Krupski WC, Bass A, Kelly AB, Marzec UM, Hanson SR, Harker LA: Heparin-resistant thrombus formation by endovascular stents in baboons: interruption by a synthetic antithrombin. *Circulation* 1990; 82:570.
15. Fulcher CA, Gardiner JE, Griffin JH, Zimmerman TS: Proteolytic inactivation of human factor VIII procoagulant protein by activated protein C and its analogy with factor V. *Blood* 1984; 63:486.
16. Broze GJ, Warren LA, Novotny WF, Higuchi DA, Girard JJ, Miletich JP: The lipoprotein-associated coagulation inhibitor that inhibits the factor VII-tissue factor complex also inhibits factor Xa: insight into its possible mechanism of action. *Blood* 1988; 71:335.
17. Schatz RA, Baim DS, Ellis LM, Goldberg S, Hirshfeld JW, Cleman MW, Cabin HS, Walker C, Stagg J, Buchbinder M, Teirstein PS, Topol EJ, Savage M, Perez JA, Curry TC, Whitworth H, Sousa JE, Tio FO, Almagor Y, Ponder R, Penn IM, Leonard B, Levine SL, Fish RD, Palmaz JC: Clinical experience with the Palmaz-Schatz coronary stent: initial results of a multicenter study. *Circulation* 1991; 83:148.
18. Roubin GS, Cannon AD, Agrawal SK, Macander PJ, Dean LS, Baxley WA, Breland J: Intracoronary stenting for acute and threatened closure complicating percutaneous transluminal coronary angioplasty. *Circulation* 1992; 85:916.
19. Serruys PW, Strauss BH, Beatt KJ, Bertrand ME, Puel J, Rickards AF, Meier B, Goy JJ, Vogt P, Kappenberger L, Sigwart U: Angiographic follow-up after placement of a self-expanding coronary-artery stent. *N Engl J Med* 1991; 324:13.
20. Furie B, Furie BC: Molecular basis of blood coagulation. *Cell* 1988; 53:505.
21. Sigwart U, Puel J, Mirkovitch V, Joffre F, Kappenberger L: Intravascular stents to prevent occlusion and restenosis after transluminal angioplasty. *N Engl J Med* 1987; 316:701.

22. Haude M, Erbel R, Straub U, Dietz U, Schatz R, Meyer J: Results of intracoronary stents for management of coronary dissection after balloon angioplasty. *Am J Cardiol* 1991;67:691.
23. Fischman DL, Savage MP, Leon MB, Hirshfeld JW Jr, Cleman MW, Teirstein P, Goldberg S: Angiographic predictors of subacute thrombosis following coronary artery stenting. *Circulation* 1991; 84(suppl II):II-588. Abstract.
24. Sutton JM, Ellis SG, Roubin GS, Muller DWM, George BS, Garratt KN, Raizner AE, Voorhees WD, Rodgers GP, Topol EJ: Differences in clinical characteristics and outcome for acute versus elective coronary artery stent placement. *Circulation* 1991; 84(suppl II):II-301. Abstract.
25. Hamm CW, Beythien C, Sievert H, Langer A, Utech A, Bauer U, Reifart N: First clinical experience with the Strecker-stent for acute coronary occlusions after PTCA. *Circulation* 1991; 84(suppl II):II-198. Abstract.
26. Nath FC, Muller DWM, Ellis SG, Chapekis AT, Zimmerman C, Topol EJ: Early thrombotic occlusion of coronary stents: frequency, predictors, therapy and clinical outcome. *Circulation* 1991; 84(suppl II):II-587. Abstract.
27. Herrmann HC, Buchbinder M, Cleman MW, Fischman D, Goldberg S, Leon MB, Teirstein P, Schatz RA, Walker CM, Hirshfeld JW Jr: Emergent use of balloon-expandable coronary artery stenting for failed PTCA. *Circulation* 1992; 86: 812–819.
28. Erbel R, Swars H, Hafner G, Haude M, Meyer J: Reduction of subacute thrombotic stent occlusion by improved anticoagulation monitoring. *Circulation* 1991; 84(suppl II):II-588. Abstract.
29. Lembo NJ, Black AJ, Roubin GS, Mufson LH, Wilentz JR, Douglas JS Jr, King SB III: Does the addition of dipyridamole to aspirin decrease acute coronary angioplasty complications? The results of a prospective randomized clincal trial. *J Am Coll Cardiol* 1988; 11(suppl A):237A. Abstract.
30. Weiss HJ: The effect of clinical dextran on platelet aggregation, adhesion, and ADP release in man: in vivo and in vitro studies. *J Lab Clin Med* 1967; 69:37.
31. Langdell RD, Adelson E, Furth FW, Crosby WH: Dextran and prolonged bleeding time. results of a sixty-gram, one-liter infusion given to 163 normal human subjects. *J Am Med Assoc* 1958; 166:346.
32. Dougherty KG, Marsh KC, Edelman SK, Gaos CM, Ferguson JJ, Leachman DR: Relationship between procedural activated clotting time and in-hospital post-PTCA outcome. *Circulation* 1990; 82(suppl III):III-189. Abstract.
33. Eisenberg PR, Sherman LA, Rich M, Schwartz D, Schectman K, Geltman EM, Sobel BE, Jaffe AS: Importance of continued activation of thrombin reflected by fibrinol peptide A to the efficacy of thrombolysis. *J Am Coll Cardiol* 1986; 7:1255.
34. Winters KJ, Santoro SA, Miletich JP, Eisenberg PR: Relative importance of thrombin compared with plasmin-mediated platelet activation in reponse to plasminogen activation with streptokinase. *Circulation* 1991; 84:1552.
35. Vaughan DE, Van Houtte E, Declerck PJ, Collen D: Streptokinase-induced platelet aggregation: prevalence and mechanism. *Circulation* 1991; 84:84.
36. Loscalzo J, Vaughn DE: Tissue plasminogen activator promotes platelet disaggregation in plasma. *J Clin Invest* 1987; 79:1749.
37. Adelman B , Michaelson AD, Loscalzo J: Plasmin effect on platelet glycoprotein Ib-von Willebrand factor interactions. *Blood* 1985; 65:32.
38. Mizuta T, Imai C: Tissue-type plasminogen activator inhibits aggregation of platelets in vitro. *Life Sci* 1988; 43:955.
39. Chapekis AT, George BS, Candela RJ: Rapid thrombus dissolution by continuous infusion of urokinase through an intracoronary perfusion wire prior to and following PTCA: results in native coronaries and patent saphenous vein grafts. *Cathet Cardiovasc Diagn* 1991; 23:89.
40. Roubin GS, Cannon AD, Agrawal SK, Macander PJ, Dean LS, Baxley WA, Breland

J: Intracoronary stenting for acute and threatened closure complicating percutaneous transluminal coronary angioplasty. *Circulation* 1992; 85:916.

41. Sigwart U, Urban P, Golf S, Kaufmann U, Imbert C, Fischer A, Kappenberger L: Emergency stenting for acute occlusion after coronary balloon angioplasty. *Circulation* 1988; 78:1121.
42. Goy J-J, Sigwart U, Vogt P, Stauffer J-C, Kaufmann U, Urban P, Kappenberger L: Long-term follow-up of the first 56 patients treated with intracoronary self-expanding stents (The Lausanne experience). *Am J Cardiol* 1991; 67:569.
43. Schomig A, Dietz R, Kubler W, Hsu E, Kranzhofer R: Outcome after emergency implantation of coronary stents. *J Am Coll Cardiol* 1992; 19(suppl A): 198A. Abstract.
44. Haude M, Erbel R, Issa H, Straub U, Swars H, Dietz U, Meyer J: Analysis of risk factors for the occurrance of subacute thrombotic events after intracoronary implantation of Palmaz-Schatz stents. *J Am Coll Cardiol* 1992; 19:77A. Abstract.
45. Dichek DA, Neville RF, Zwiebel JA, Freeman SM, Leon MB, Anderson WF: Seeding of intravascular stents with genetically engineered endothelial cells. *Circulation* 1989;80:1347.
46. Nabel EG, Plautz G, Nabel GJ: Site-specific gene expression in vivo by direct gene transfer into the arterial wall. *Science* 1990; 249:1285.
47. Lim CS, Chapman GD, Gammon RS, Muhlestein JB, Bauman RP, Stack RS, Swain JL: Direct in vivo gene transfer into the coronary and peripheral vasculatures of the intact dog. *Circulation* 1991; 83:2007.
48. Bier JD, Zalesky P, Sasken H, Williams DO: A new bioabsorbable intravascular stent: in vitro assessment of hemodynamic and morphometric characteristics. *Circulation* 1991; 84(suppl Il):II-197a. Abstract.
49. Schwartz RS, Huber KC, Edwards WD, Taswell HF, Canmrud AR, Jorgenson MA, Holmes DR Jr: Native fibrin film as a biocompatible, absorbable material for intracoronary stent implant and drug delivery. *J Am Coll Cardiol* 1992; 19:171a. Abstract.

III

Clinical Indications

CHAPTER 4

Coronary Artery Stenting for Intimal Dissection

Michael P. Savage
David L. Fischman
Andrew Zalewski
Sheldon Goldberg

A major limitation of standard balloon angioplasty is the occurrence of abrupt vessel closure in the immediate periprocedural period. When this complication occurs, the risks of death, myocardial infarction, and urgent coronary artery bypass grafting increase dramatically.[1] Prior studies have shown that intimal dissection is an important mechanism responsible for abrupt closure.[2] The purpose of this chapter is to describe the efficacy of a new technology, the Palmaz-Schatz balloon-expandable stent[3] in resolving the problem of balloon-induced intimal disruption.

Morbidity and Mortality of Standard Percutaneous Transluminal Coronary Angioplasty

Previous investigators have established morbidity and mortality rates for elective percutaneous transluminal coronary angioplasty (PTCA).[4] In a large study of more than 3000 consecutive patients undergoing PTCA by three experienced operators at Emory University Hospital, all in-hospital complications were prospectively recorded. Major ischemic complications defined as death, myocardial infarction, or the need for urgent coronary artery bypass grafting were noted in 145 patients or 4.1%. By far, the strongest independent predictor of a major complication was the intraprocedural appearance of an intimal dissection. Intimal dissection occurred in 894/3099 patients.(29%) In these patients, 93 (10.4%) developed a major complication compared with only 35 of 2205 (1.6%) patients without evidence of an intimal dissection ($P < 0.0001$)

From: Herrmann HC, Hirshfeld JW, eds. *Clinical Use of the Palmaz-Schatz Intracoronary Stent.* Futura Publishing Company, Inc., Mount Kisco, NY, © 1993.

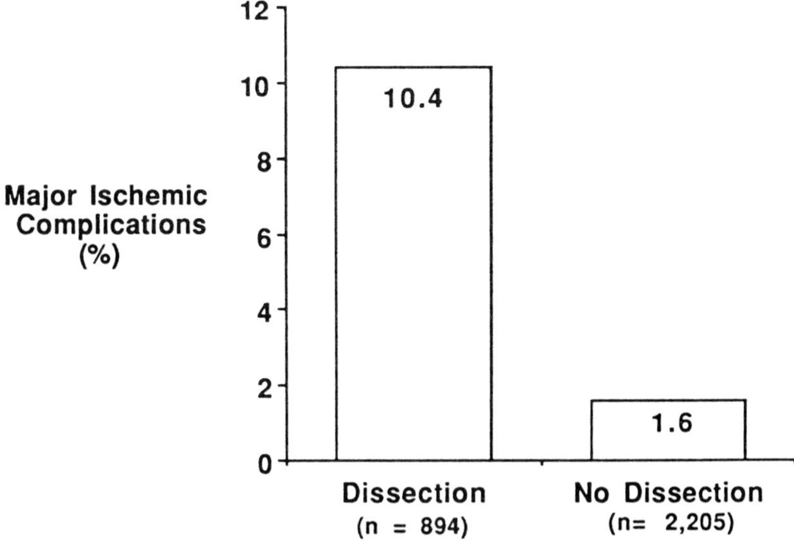

Figure 1: *The incidence of major in-hospital complications in patients with and without intimal dissection after standard PTCA. Major complications included death, myocardial infarction, and urgent coronary bypass grafting. Note the 6.5-fold increase in these events if intimal dissection occurred during the angioplasty procedure. (Adapted from[4]).*

(Fig. 1). Therefore, the development of an intimal tear was associated with a 6.5-fold increase in the risk of a major ischemic event.[4] Certain baseline angiographic and clinical variables have been associated with an increased risk for intimal disruption and subsequent vessel closure; these include lesion complexity and eccentricity, lesion length, branch or bend points and calcification.[4,5]

Role of Stenting for Intimal Dissection

Since intimal tearing is the most frequent operative mechanism for major complications, the role of an intracoronary scaffold in the form of a metallic stent has been examined as an approach for sealing intimal flaps and enlarging the coronary lumen after balloon-induced intimal disruption. The mechanism by which stenting exerts its beneficial effect in this circumstance is illustrated in Figure 2.[6] An atherosclerotic human cadaver coronary artery which has been subjected to post-mortem balloon dilatation has developed an intimal and medial disruption with a tissue flap that impinges on the vessel lumen (Fig. 2A). A similar coronary artery is depicted in the lower panel; the latter vessel was first dilated with a standard angioplasty balloon and also developed an intimal and medial tear (light arrow). A stent was then inserted; the deployed struts of this device are seen on end in this cross section (heavy arrows). The

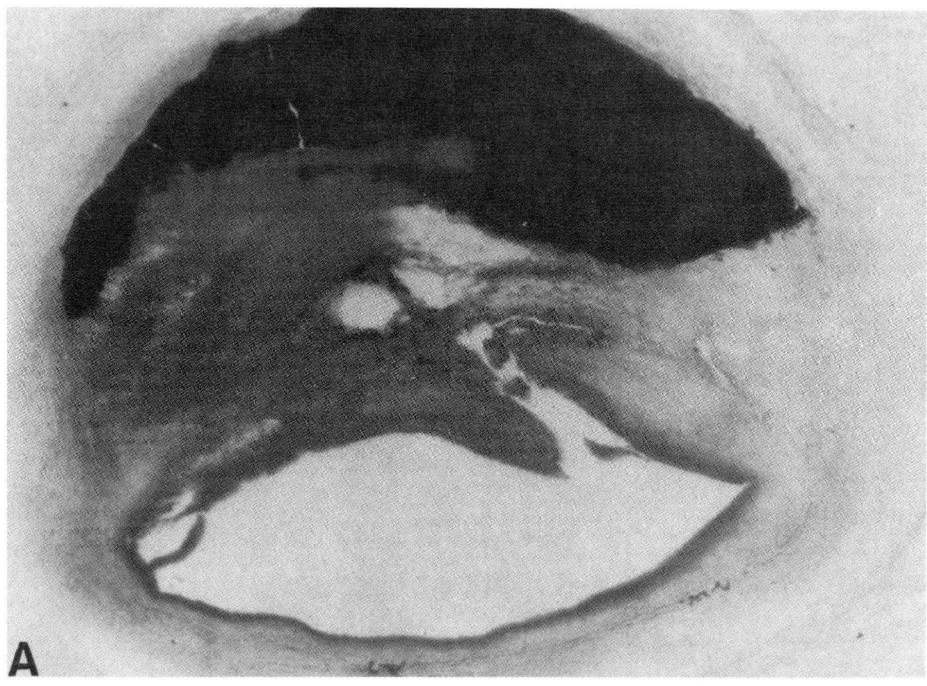

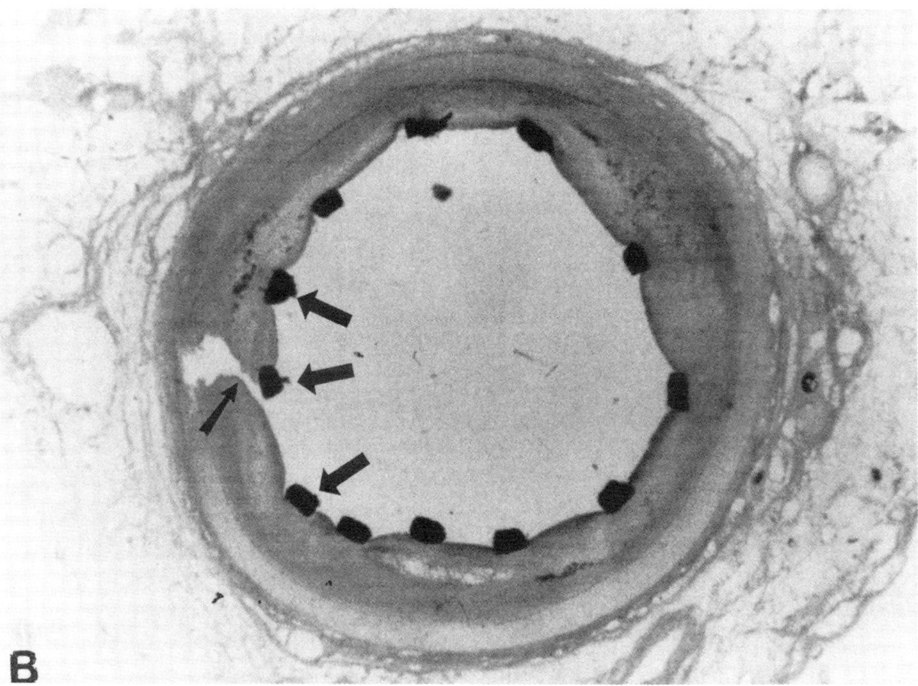

Figure 2: *The mechanism of stent efficacy in resolving intimal dissections. In 2A, a cadaver coronary artery subject to balloon angioplasty is seen. Note severe intimal dissection with a tissue flap compromising the vessel lumen. A stented coronary artery is shown in 2B; note the intimal-medial tear (small arrow) successfully sealed by stent struts (heavy arrows). (Adapted from,*[6] *with permission).*

intimal-medial dissection is sealed by the device, with resolution of the protruding flap and a large smooth coronary lumen (Fig. 2B).

In order to test the hypothesis that coronary artery stenting would be successful in sealing intimal dissections in the clinical setting, we evaluated the Palmaz-Schatz stent using qualitative and quantitative coronary analyses.[7]

Methods

Patients

Eighty-four consecutive patients who underwent stenting and had subsequent coronary analysis formed the basis of the study. All had the following inclusion criteria: presence of single-vessel disease with the target lesion greater than 70% by visual estimate, objective evidence of myocardial ischemia, and preserved left ventricular function with an ejection fraction of greater than or equal to 50%. All patients gave informed consent to protocols approved by the Institutional Review Boards of the eight participating centers.

All patients underwent angioplasty using standard over-the-wire steerable systems. After PTCA, an exchange wire was left in place in the distal coronary artery and the stent was delivered over a standard balloon. The patients were given aspirin, 325 mg per day, and a calcium antagonist for greater than or equal to 48 hours before stent placement. Heparin, 10,000 U, was given intravenously, followed by an infusion that was adjusted to maintain the activated clotting time greater than 300 seconds. Low-molecular weight dextran was started 3 hours prior to the procedure and infused over 10 to 20 hours (1 liter). Warfarin was administered after the procedure, and heparin was continued until the prothrombin time was 16 to 18 seconds. Anticoagulation with warfarin was continued for 1 month. Aspirin was continued indefinitely.

Quantitative Analysis

Cine frames at baseline, after PTCA and after stent placement, were selected by the panel of angiographers for quantitative lesion measurement. Paired orthogonal views were utilized whenever possible. Analyses were carried out using a computer-based edge detection system.[8,9] The selected frames were projected using a 35-mm cine-viewer which was optically coupled to a videocamera. The signal was digitized at 512 × 512 × 8-bit resolution onto a digital angiographic computer. The images were magnified fourfold and the region of interest was defined by the operator. The vessel contour was then defined by the computer using a previously validated edge detection algorithm. Quantitative measurements including minimal lumen diameter and stenosis length were determined by using the guiding catheter as a scaling factor. An

Table 1.
Classification of Intimal Dissection

Type	Grade	Definition
No dissection	0	No intimal disruption
Simple dissection	1A	Intraluminal linear defect
	1B	Extraluminal cap extravasation
Complex dissection	2A	Nonlinear spiral defect
	2B	Luminal defect with multiple irregular borders
	2C	Obstructive dissection

average of the proximal and distal segments outside the stented region was used to calculate the reference-diameter and percent-diameter stenosis.

Qualitative Analysis

All angiograms from stented patients of multicenter-stent investigators were reviewed at a core angiographic laboratory established at Thomas Jefferson University Hospital. Coronary arteriography was performed in the baseline control state, after standard PTCA, and after implantation of the stents. Three experienced angiographers interpreted all films, and detailed morphologic analyses were performed. Intimal dissections were classified as follows: (Table 1): grade 0, no dissection; grade 1, simple dissection consisting of an intraluminal linear defect (IA) or an extraluminal "cap extravasation" (IB); or grade 2, defined as a complex dissection consisting of a nonlinear spiral defect (2A), a luminal defect with multiple irregular borders (2B), or an obstructive defect (2C).

Lesions were also characterized for the following factors known to be associated with reduced primary success[10]: eccentricity, calcification, thrombus, plaque ulceration, and vessel tortuosity. An eccentric lesion was defined as one in which the stenotic lumen was located within one-half of the original lumen in at least one projection. Intracoronary thrombus was defined as an intraluminal filling defect surrounded by dye or as a total obstruction with a convex border or prolonged contrast staining, or both. A complex, ulcerated stenosis was defined as an eccentric lesion with a narrow neck associated with an overhanging edge or irregular borders. Diffuse disease was defined as multiple lumen narrowings in adjacent nonstented segments of the coronary artery. A tortuous lesion was one located on a bend of greater than or equal to 45° within the segment to be stented.

Results

One hundred-six stents were placed for 90 lesions in the 84 patients. The frequency of balloon-induced intimal dissection is shown in Figure 3.[7] Thirty-

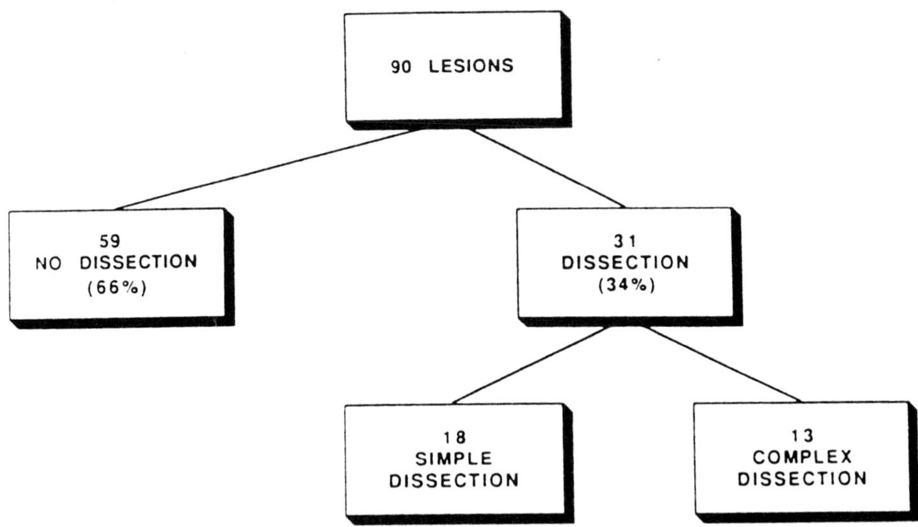

Figure 3: *The incidence of intimal dissection after standard balloon dilatation in a consecutive series of patients subsequently treated with stents. Some degree of intimal disruption occurred in 34% of lesions. (Adapted from,[7] with permission).*

one dissections developed in the 90 dilated lesions (34%). Of these 31 dissections, 18 were classified as simple, grade 1 tears (58%), and 13 were classified as complex, grade 2 dissections (42%). The baseline preangioplasty qualitative and quantitative characteristics of the 90 stented lesions are shown in Table 2. There were no differences between the groups with and without dissection with respect to lesion location. However, lesion complexity was noted twice as frequently in the group that developed intimal tears. In addition, lesion eccentricity was slightly, although not statistically, more frequent in the dissection group. These stents were placed in relatively large vessels with discrete stenoses; the average vessel diameter was 3.2 ± 0.5 mm and the mean lesion length was 8.6 ± 5.0 mm.

The effect of stent placement on the intimal dissection grade is illustrated in Figure 4. Of the 18 lesions which developed simple (grade 1) dissections after balloon dilatation, 16 were reduced to grade 0. Of the 13 lesions that developed complex (grade 2) dissections after standard balloon angioplasty, 11 were reduced to grade 0, and two complex disruptions were reduced to grade 1 tears. Therefore, stent placement completely resolved intimal disruption in 27/31 instances or 87%. Importantly, in no case did a patient leave the catheterization suite with a complex dissection after stent placement.

The results of quantitative analysis for the 31 lesions that developed intimal disruption were as follows (Fig. 5). At baseline, the mean-percent stenosis was 77 ± 17%; after PTCA the average-percent stenosis was 47 ± 17%; following stent implantation the residual stenosis was significantly improved to 14 ± 10%.

Table 2.
Comparison of Baseline Characteristics of 90 Coronary Lesions With and Without Dissection After Balloon Angioplasty*

Variable	*Dissection*	*No Dissection*	*p Value*
No. of lesions	31	59	
Lesion site			NS
LMCA	3	0	
LAD	39	34	
LCx	13	7	
RCA	45	57	
SVG	0	2	
Lesion morphology			
Eccentric	56	47	NS
Calcification	10	15	NS
Bend $\geq$ 45°	3	3	NS
Complex	54	29	< 0.05
Diffuse	25	23	NS
Thrombus	17	7	NS
Percent-diameter stenosis (mean ± SD)	77 ± 17	72 ± 15	NS
Reference vessel (mm)	3.3 ± 0.4	3.2 ± 0.5	NS
Lesion length (mm)	9.8 ± 6.6	8.1 ± 3.9	NS

* Unless otherwise indicated, data reported are percents. LAD = left anterior descending coronary artery; LCx = left circumflex coronary artery; LMCA = left main coronary artery; RCA = right coronary artery; SVG = saphenous vein graft.

The clinical outcomes of the patients who developed dissections were notable for the occurrence of stent thrombosis in only one instance. In this patient, sudden closure occurred 12 days after stent implantation; this patient was managed by intracoronary thrombolysis and urgent redilation.

Illustrative Cases

Case 1

A 63-year-old male had class IV angina of one week's duration. After maximal medical therapy, the patient underwent coronary angiography. The baseline coronary arteriogram in the left anterior oblique view is shown in Figure 6A. Note that in the baseline state there is a complex, eccentric stenosis, which represents a high-risk lesion for standard balloon angioplasty (Fig. 6B). Quantitative angiography showed that the lesion was 9.2 mm in length, and there was a 76%–diameter stenosis narrowing. After standard angioplasty, there was a suboptimal result due to intimal disruption and elastic recoil, and there was no significant change in the diameter stenosis.

Because of the suboptimal result in this high-risk lesion, we placed a single Palmaz-Schatz stent. There was marked improvement in the lumen diameter, with a 0% stenosis present at the end of the procedure (Fig. 6C). This patient has remained asymptomatic and the 6- and 12-month follow-up by angiogram showed no evidence of restenosis.

Case 2

A 73-year-old woman with unstable angina of 10 days duration was treated with aspirin, heparin, β-blockers, and nitrates. Cardiac catheterization demonstrated a severe stenosis in the midportion of the left circumflex coronary artery (Figure 7A). The intima appeared disrupted, and there was a hazy appearance of the vessel just distal to the most severe luminal narrowing (arrow). Quantitative coronary analysis of the baseline angiogram showed a significant stenosis of 69%.

The patient underwent standard percutaneous transluminal angioplasty with a suboptimal result as noted in Figure 7B. There is a simple linear coronary artery dissection and the lumen is compromised with a residual diameter stenosis of 46%. Therefore, the patient underwent placement of a single Palmaz-Schatz stent, which resulted in an excellent angiographic outcome (Fig. 7C). The intimal tear is completely resolved associated with improvement in the residual narrowing to a 12%–diameter stenosis after stent implantation.

This patient has remained asymptomatic and a 6-month angiographic follow-up showed continued patency of the artery without evidence of restenosis.

Case 3

A 65-year-old man developed unstable angina and was treated with a full medical regimen including aspirin, heparin, calcium antagonists, and β-blockers. Subsequent coronary angiography showed a severe, complex lesion in the midleft anterior descending coronary artery (Fig. 8A). There was severe intimal disruption, a cap dissection was present, and a flap compromised the coronary lumen. Quantitative angiographic analysis showed a 75%–diameter narrowing. The patient had attempted balloon angioplasty, but this resulted in no change in the appearance of this lesion. The dissection cap continued to be present along with the intimal flap compromising the lumen. Therefore, a single Palmaz-Schatz stent was inserted.

The stent-balloon assembly was easily passed through the disrupted coronary segment and a test injection (Fig. 8B) showed that the stent spanned the entire length of the disrupted coronary artery (note balloon markers bracketing the stent).

Figure 8C shows the results after stent placement. There is complete resolution of the dissection and marked improvement in the diameter stenosis. Quantitative coronary analysis showed a 16%–diameter stenosis after stent implantation. This patient has remained asymptomatic and the 6-month angiogram showed no evidence of restenosis.

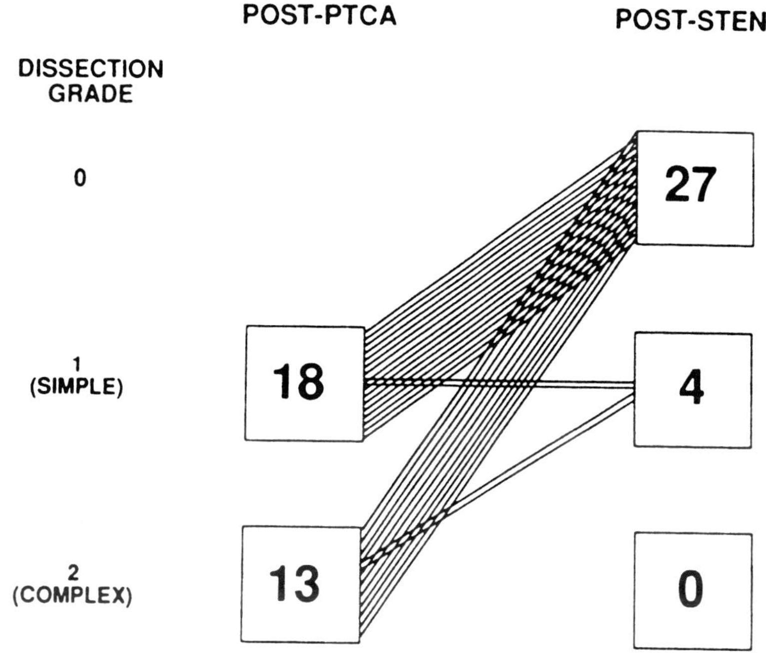

Figure 4: *The results of stent placement on initial dissection grade. Complete resolution of dissection occurred in 87%. In no case did a patient leave the catheterization suite with a complex dissection. (Adapted from,[7] with permission).*

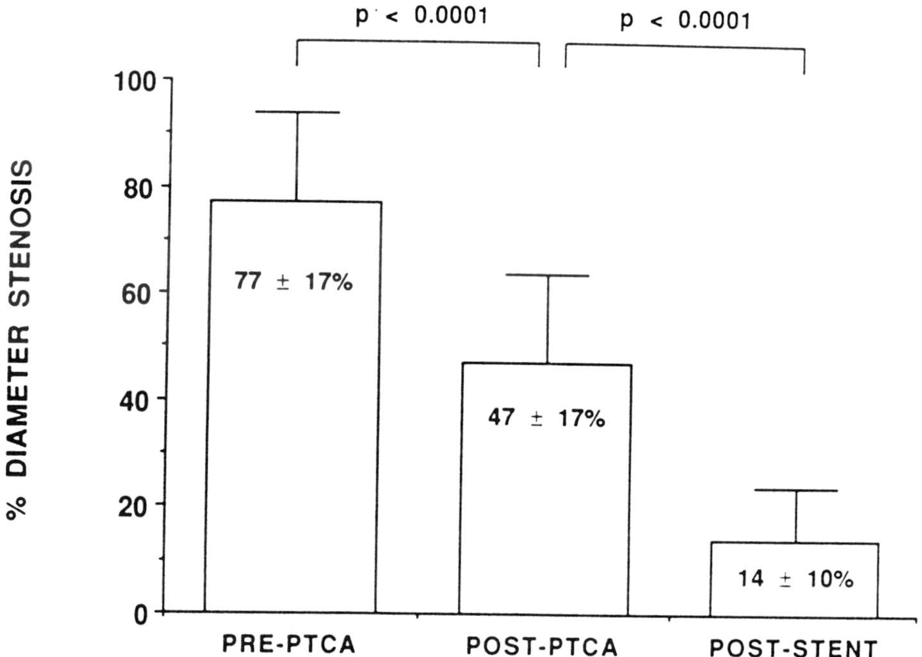

Figure 5: *The results of stenting on percent-diameter stenosis for patients in whom intimal dissection developed. There is a dramatic improvement in the degree of luminal narrowing for this group. (Adapted from,[7] with permission).*

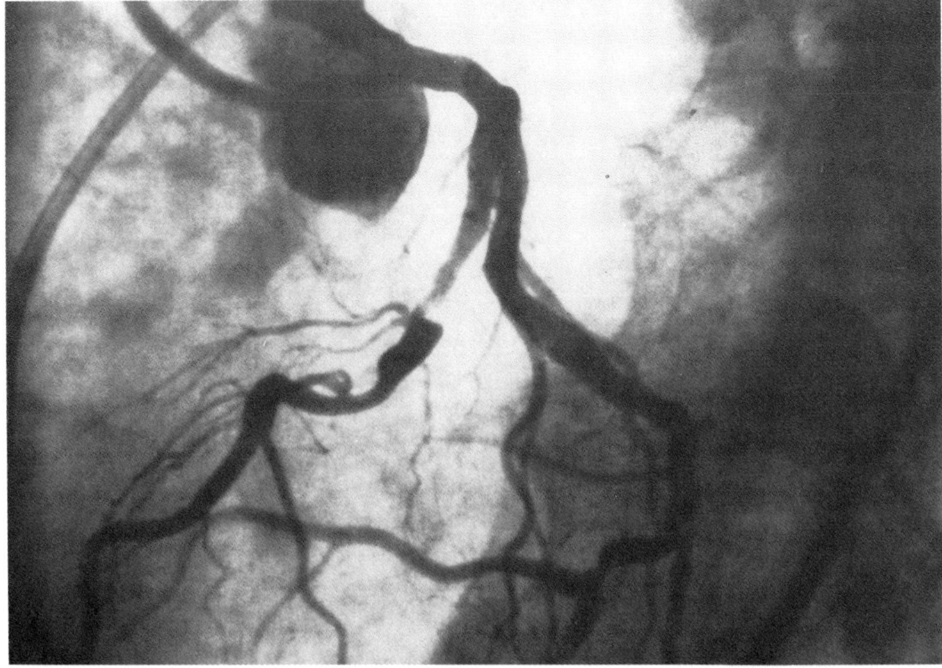

Figure 6A: *Baseline left coronary arteriogram in left anterior oblique views. Note the complex, eccentric stenosis. This is a typical high-risk lesion for standard PTCA. Also note there is no visible thrombus present, and the lesion is relatively discrete.*

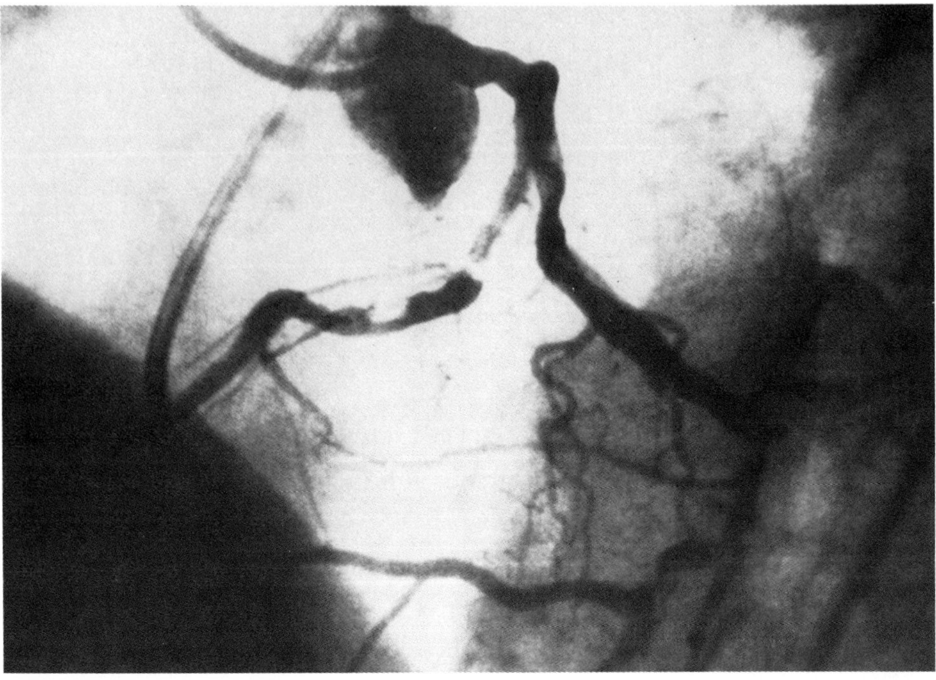

Figure 6B: *Result after standard PTCA. Views as in Fig. 6A. The result is suboptimal due to intimal disruption and elastic recoil.*

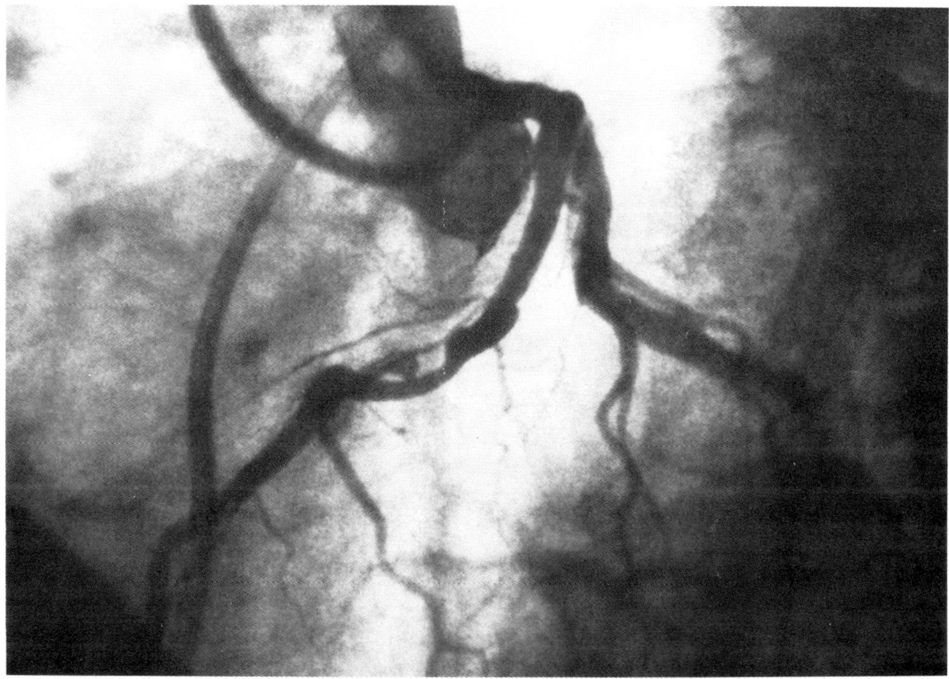

Figure 6C: *Results after placement of a single Palmaz-Schatz stent. Note the marked improvement in lumen diameter and the resolution of the intimal dissection.*

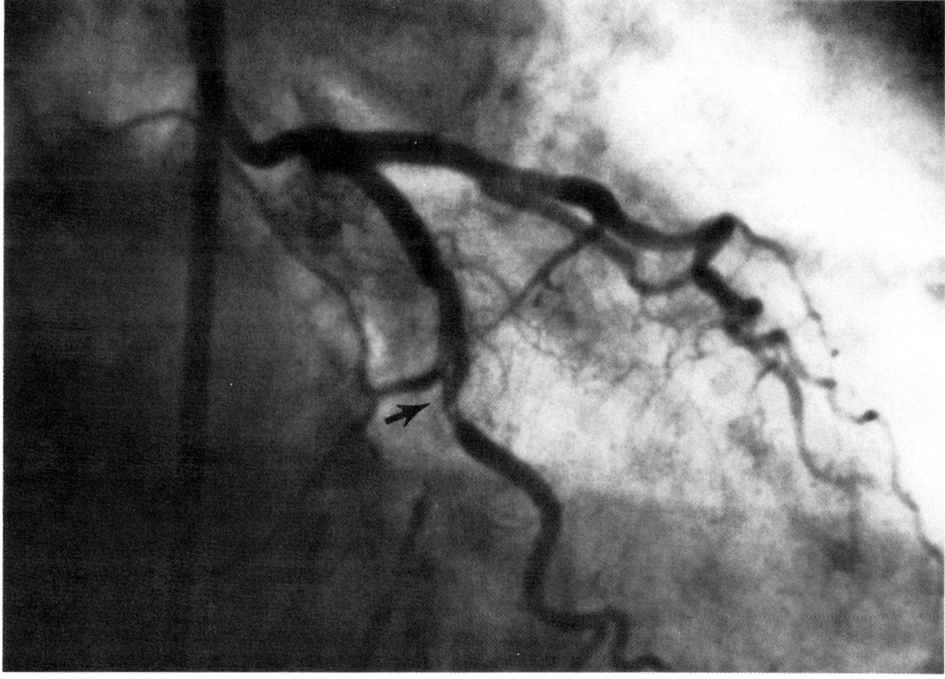

Figure 7A: *Baseline left coronary angiogram in the right anterior oblique view. Note the intimal disruption and hazy appearance of the left circumflex coronary artery.*

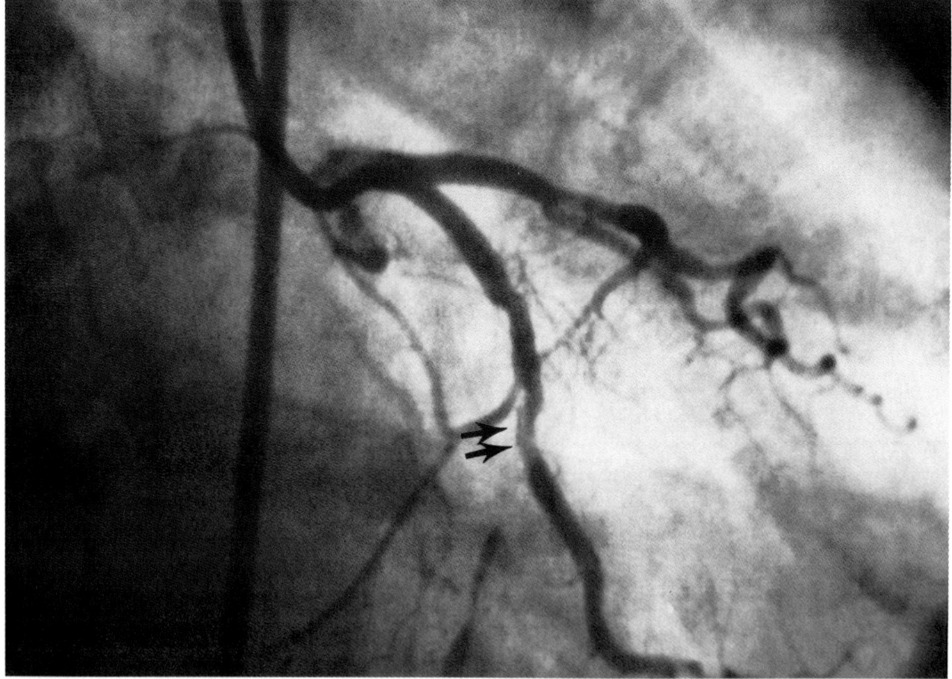

Figure 7B: *Result after standard PTCA; the dissection is still evident and the lumen is compromised.*

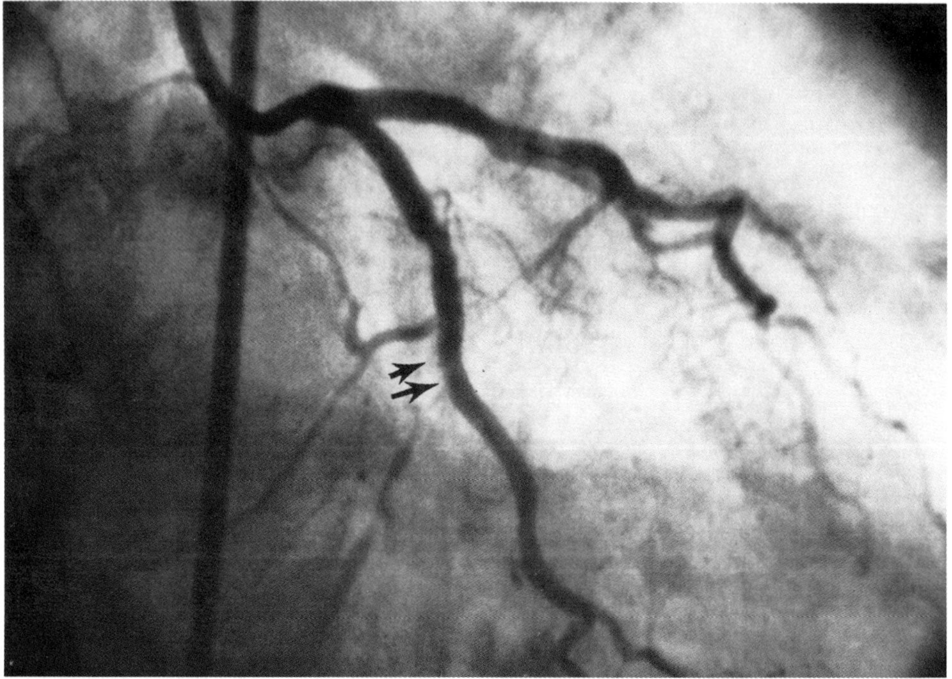

Figure 7C: *Result after placement of a single Palmaz-Schatz stent. The dissection is completely resolved and the lumen diameter improved.*

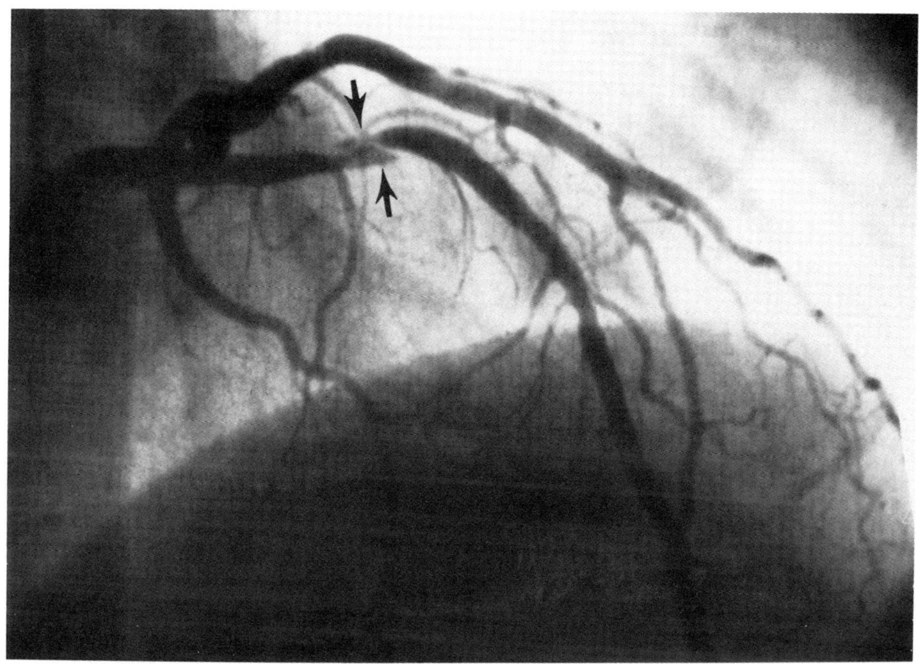

Figure 8A: *Baseline left coronary angiogram in the right anterior oblique projection from a patient who underwent standard balloon angioplasty of the left anterior descending coronary artery. Note the severe intimal disruption, cap dissection, and compromised lumen. This is a complex, grade 2 dissection.*

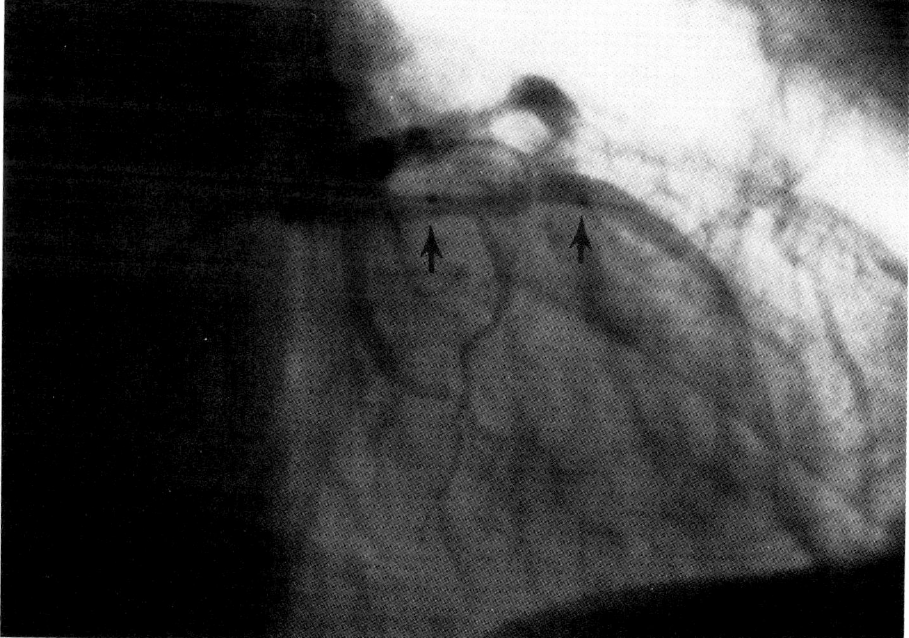

Figure 8B: *A test injection with stent-balloon assembly placed across the disrupted coronary segment. The ends of the unexpanded stent are delineated by the markers (arrows). The operator can now be assured that the stent covers the entire segment.*

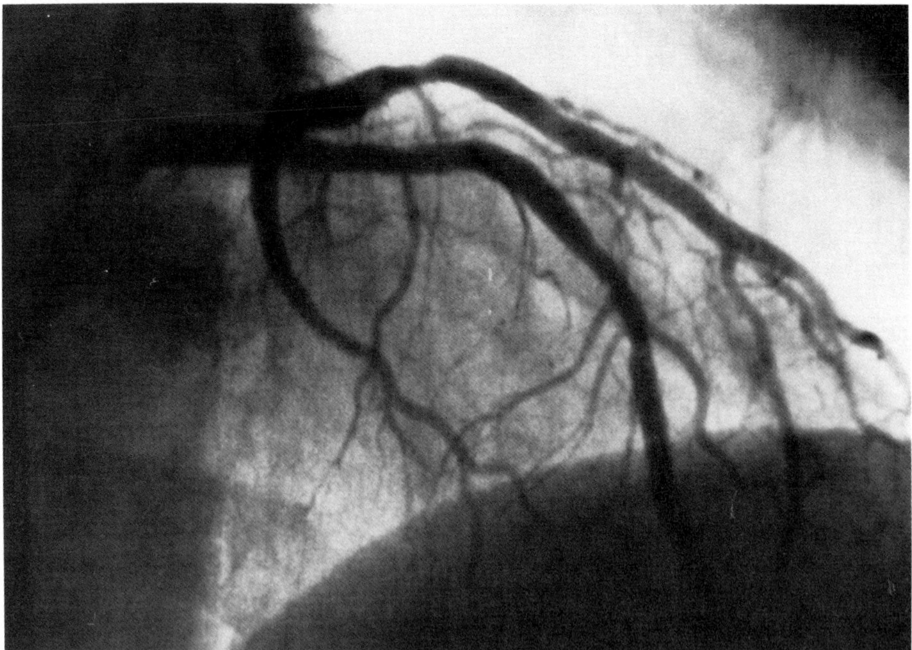

Figure 8C: *Result after stent placement. There is complete resolution of the dissection and marked improvement in the percent-diameter stenosis.*

Discussion

The results of studies performed by the multicenter-stent investigators have established that the Palmaz-Schatz stent is an effective device for resolving intimal tears that develop after standard balloon angioplasty. Since certain morphologic lesion characteristics have been shown to be associated with a higher rate of intimal disruption and subsequent vessel closure, the planned use of the stent for these types of lesions may lead to improved primary angioplasty outcomes compared with standard balloon dilatation. However, data to confirm this hypothesis are not yet available.

In our center, we have prepared patients with high-risk lesion morphology for possible stent implantation. If we encounter patients with discrete, complex, or eccentric lesions which do not contain thrombus, we have proceeded with standard PTCA; if the result is satisfactory after the procedure, patients are followed with standard post-PTCA protocols. If an intimal tear develops, attempts are made to seal the flap by the use of prolonged inflations with an autoperfusion catheter, if necessary. If this maneuver fails to adequately resolve the intimal disruption, we proceed with stent placement. It should be noted that discrete disruptions are more favorable than long spiral dissections for stent placement. Every effort is made to completely span the disrupted region. It is especially important not to leave a dissection outside the stented segment, as this may lead to subsequent stent thrombosis.[11] Also, we do not favor stent placement as anything more than a bridge to surgery if an intracoronary thrombus is present after stent placement. This finding also places patients at a substantially higher risk for thrombotic closure at the stented site.[11]

Certain important clinical limitations of coronary artery stenting should be emphasized. First is the problem of thrombosis, which occurs in approximately 5% of patients who have stents placed.[11] This complication develops an average of 6 days after the procedure (range 1–23 days) and may frequently result in myocardial infarction. While vigorous anticoagulation decreases the incidence of this problem, the risk may be higher when the stent is placed in the unstable environment of an acutely disrupted vessel.[12] Second, because of the need for the use of dextran, heparin, and the combination of aspirin and warfarin, there is an increased risk of bleeding and groin complications.[7] These factors also prolong the hospital stay compared with standard balloon angioplasty.[13]

In summary, our studies have shown a salutary angiographic effect of coronary stent placement in resolving intimal dissections in almost 90% of cases. In patients who developed intimal dissections, the scaffolding effect of the stent resulted in an improvement of the mean-diameter stenosis from a suboptimal 47% after PTCA to 14% after stenting. Further studies will be required to assess the clinical efficacy of stent implantation for patients with unfavorable lesion characteristics or patients who develop serious intimal disruptions after standard PTCA.

REFERENCES

1. Detre KM, Holmes DR, Holubkov MS, Cowley MJ, Bourassa MG, Faxon DP, Dorros GR, Bentivoglio LG, Kent KM, Myler RK, Coinvestigators of the National Heart, Lung, and Blood Institute's Percutaneous Transluminal Coronary Angioplasty Registry: Incidence and consequences of periprocedural occlusion. The 1985–1986 National Heart, Lung, and Blood Institute Registry. *Circulation* 1990; 82:739–750.
2. Waller BF: "Crackers, breakers, stretchers, drillers, scrapers, shavers, burners, welders and melters": the future treatment of atherosclerotic coronary artery disease? A clinical-morphologic assessment. *J Am Coll Cardiol* 1989; 13:969–987.
3. Schatz RA, Baim DS, Leon M: Clinical experience with the Palmaz-Schatz coronary stent: Initial results of a multi-center study. *Circulation* 1991;83:148–161.
4. Bredlau CE, Roubin GS, Leimgruber PP, Douglas JS, King SB, Gruentzig AR: In hospital morbidity and mortality in patients undergoing elective coronary angioplasty. *Circulation* 1985; 72(5):1044–1052.
5. Ellis SG, Roubin GS, King SB, Dourglas JS, Weintraub WS, Thomas RG, Cox WR: Angiographic and clinical predictors of acute closure after native vessel coronary angioplasty. *Circulation* 1988; 77(2):371–379.
6. Schatz RA: A view of vascular stents. *Circulation* 1989; 79:445–457.
7. Fischman DF, Savage MP, Leon MB, Schatz RA, Ellis SG, Cleman MW, Teirstein P, Walker CM, Bailey S, Hirshfeld JW, Goldberg S: Effect of intracoronary stenting on intimal dissection after balloon angioplasty: results of quantitative and qualitative coronary analysis. *J Am Coll Cardiol* 1991; 18:1445–1451.
8. LeFree MT, Simon SB, Mancini GBJ, Vogel RA: Digital radiographic assessment

of coronary arterial geometric diameter and videodensitometric cross-sectional area. *Proc Soc Photo-optical Instru Engi* 1986; 626:334–341.

9. Mancini GBJ, Simon SB, McGillem MJ, LeFree MT, Friedman HZ, Vogel RA: Automated quantitative coronary arteriography: morphologic and physiologic validation in vivo of a rapid digital angiographic method. *Circulation* 1987; 75:452–460.
10. Ryan TJ, Faxon DP, Gunnar RM, Kennedy JW, King SB, Loop FD, Peterson KL, Reeves TJ, Williams DO, Winters WL: Guidelines for percutaneous transluminal coronary angioplasty: a report of the American College of Cardiology/American Heart Association Task Force on assessment of diagnostic and therapeutic cardiovascular procedures. *J Am Coll Cardiol* 1988; 12:529–545.
11. Fischman DL, Savage MP, Leon MB, Hirshfeld JW Jr, Cleman MW, Teirstein P, Goldberg S: Angiographic predictors of subacute thrombosis following coronary artery stenting. *Circulation* 1991; 84(II):558.
12. Herrmann HC, Buchbinder M, Cleman MW, Fischman D, Goldberg S, Leon MB, Schatz RA, Teirstein P, Walker CM, Hirshfeld JW Jr: Emergent use of balloon expandable coronary artery stenting for failed PTCA. *Circulation* 1992; 86: 812–819.
13. Dick RJ, Burek KA, Muller DW, Topol EJ: The incremental costs associated with the use of new percutaneous coronary devices. *Circulation* 1990;82(III):71.

CHAPTER 5

Restenosis Following Palmaz-Schatz Coronary Artery Stenting

Joseph P. Carrozza, Jr.
Donald S. Baim

Historical Perspectives

In 1979, Gruentzig reported the first series of patients treated with percutaneous transluminal coronary angioplasty,[1] heralding a new era in myocardial revascularization. Tempering the initial enthusiasm for this technique, however, was the observation that recurrent stenoses occurred in a significant fraction of patients,[2] within 6 months of successful dilation. Improvements in equipment design and operator experience have led to higher success and lower complication rates,[3] but the rate of restenosis has remained 30% to 40%.[2,4–9] In an effort to reduce the incidence of restenosis, a number of trials have examined various pharmacotherapies including antiplatelet agents,[10] anticoagulants,[10,11] calcium-channel antagonists,[12] ω-3-fatty acids,[13] and corticosteroids.[14] To date, however, no agent or class of agents has definitively reduced the incidence of restenosis. More recently, several newer technologies, such as laser-balloon angioplasty,[15] directional coronary atherectomy,[16] and coronary stenting[17,18] have entered evaluation to determine their efficacy in reducing the incidence of restenosis. This chapter will discuss the incidence and mechanisms responsible for restenosis after balloon angioplasty and coronary artery stenting, as well as the management of this problem.

Problems in Evaluating Restenosis

Uncertain Definition of Restenosis

One of the major issues complicating analysis of restenosis has been the lack of a single-consensus definition. While some studies have relied upon

From: Herrmann HC, Hirshfeld JW, eds. *Clinical Use of the Palmaz-Schatz Intracoronary Stent.* Futura Publishing Company, Inc., Mount Kisco, NY, © 1993.

Table 1.
Commonly Used Definitions of Restenosis

	Definition	*Reference*
NHLBI I[2]	≥ 30% increase in post-PTCA MLD at follow-up	2
NHLBI II[2]	< 50% stenosis post-PTCA increasing to ≥ 70% at follow-up	2
NHLBI III[2]	Follow-up stenosis within 10% of pre-PTCA stenosis	2
NHLBI IV[2]	Loss of ≥ 50% of gain post-PTCA	2
Loss ≥ 0.72 mm[7]	Loss of ≥ 0.72 mm in MLD at follow-up	7
≥ 50% diameter stenosis[20]	Follow-up stenosis ≥ 50%	20

NHLBI = National Heart, Lung and Blood Institute.
MLD = minimum lumen diameter.

clinical end points (such as recurrent angina or exercise-induced ischemia[19]) as surrogates for restenosis, most major studies have defined restenosis angiographically. Six different angiographic definitions of restenosis have been proposed[2,7,20] (Table 1). The advantages and disadvantages of these definitions were recently summarized by Califf.[21] Since stents are usually placed in vessels greater than 2.75 mm, a loss of 0.72 mm at follow-up may not cause a flow-limiting stenosis; we therefore do not support the use of a 0.72 mm-loss as a definition of in-stent restenosis. A definition based on late-percent stenosis is preferred, but the incidence of restenosis depends upon the exact cutoff (50% or 60%) chosen.[2,7,8,17] To avoid problems relative to choosing a specific cutoff, our group has proposed viewing restenosis in a definition-independent way, using a *cumulative distribution function plot*[22] (Fig. 1). While each of these traditional definitions has its own advantages, they all are limited by their characterization of restenosis as a dichotomous (all or none) outcome. This may be appropriate for clinical decision-making (e.g., deciding whether to perform revascularization), but it fails to account for the ubiquitous biological process of intimal hyperplasia triggered by the arterial injury that accompanies any intervention.[23,24]

Kuntz has shown that the late-lumen diameter after stenting follows a Gaussian distribution, and that it is best represented as a continuous variable. Based on this concept, a geometric model of restenosis has been proposed[24] that divides it into constituent parts: acute gain and late loss. Acute gain refers to the increase in minimum lumen diameter produced by the intervention. Late loss refers to the reduction in follow-up lumen diameter produced by restenosis. This model provides an important technique for evaluating the efficacy of a new coronary intervention such as the Palmaz-Schatz stent. For example, it can be used to determine whether a reduction in incidence of restenosis that follows an intervention is due to a larger postprocedure lumen diameter, (i.e., increased acute gain), or a reduction in subsequent intimal hyperplasia, (i.e., by decreasing late loss).

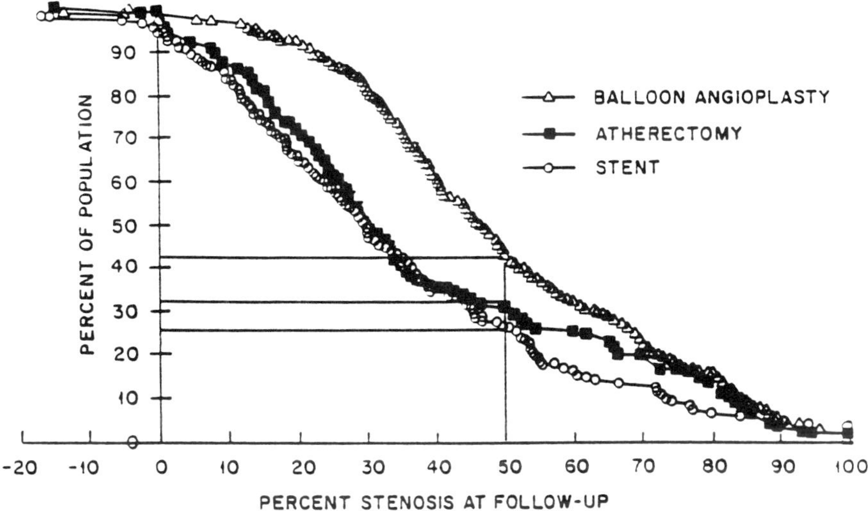

Figure 1: *Restenosis following three coronary interventions is analyzed using a cumulative distribution function plot. Restenosis as a binary event can be viewed using multiple cutoffs (with permission from the Journal of the American College of Cardiology).*

Incomplete Angiographic Follow-Up

Ideally, studies of angiographic restenosis should be performed in cohorts, with complete angiographic follow-up. Realistically, 100% angiographic follow-up is almost never achieved in large studies. In fact, angiographic follow-up rates typically range from 55% to 98%.[25] If angiographic follow-up rates fall below 70% to 80%, the problem of selection bias becomes apparent. For example, asymptomatic patients are more likely to refuse repeat angiography than are patients with recurrent symptoms, which falsely raises the apparent incidence of restenosis among the restudied population.[21] In order to minimize this effect, studies defining restenosis by angiographic criteria should have at least 75% angiographic follow-up performed 3 to 6 months following the intervention.

Different Patient Populations

The incidence of restenosis following percutaneous transluminal coronary angioplasty (PTCA) has historically been quoted to be approximately 30%,[2] but restenosis rates as low as 24%[26] and as high as 44%[8] have been reported. Even allowing for differences in definition, it is clear that restenosis rates differ depending upon patient, lesion, and procedural variables.[2,9,27–29] Given the strong dependence of restenosis rates upon these factors, it becomes evident that direct comparisons of restenosis rates in different trials may be difficult.

In order to control for these confounding variables, prospective, randomized trials have been instituted to determine the efficacy of various interventions. Califf has summarized some of the salient problems with many of these trials, including differing definitions of restenosis, variable rates and intervals of angiographic follow-up, false-positive studies resulting from multiple comparisons, and false-negative studies secondary to inadequate sample size.[21] These limitations are particularly relevant when evaluating the efficacy of a new intervention such as stenting, since large, prospective trials comparing stenting with balloon angioplasty have not been completed.

Pathophysiology of Restenosis

The anatomical and functional disturbances associated with balloon angioplasty have been well characterized based on data from post-mortem,[30] angioscopic,[31] atherectomy,[32] and experimental studies.[23,33]. Balloon dilatation is often accompanied by vessel deformation and intimal tearing[31] that triggers intimal platelet and thrombin deposition. Using quantitative angiography, Rensing has shown that immediate elastic recoil erodes up to 50% of the luminal cross-sectional area present during balloon inflation.[34] Vasoconstriction may further reduce the gain achieved with balloon angioplasty.[35] These processes may contribute to restenosis by limiting the magnitude of acute gain achieved during balloon dilation.

Within several days, mechanical stretch and enhanced production of growth factors including platelet-derived growth factor stimulate smooth muscle cell proliferation and migration into the intima. This hyperplastic response peaks at 4 to 12 weeks[23] and accounts for the observation that clinical restenosis usually occurs within this time period.[8] Experimental and angiographic data obtained following a variety of new coronary interventions such as stenting, directional atherectomy, and laser-balloon angioplasty, show that intimal hyperplasia appears to be a ubiquitous event following all forms of arterial injury.[23,24] Quantification of the late loss due to intimal hyperplasia provides a more accurate reflection of this process than the traditional view of restenosis as a dichotomous all-or-none outcome.

Restenosis Rates and the Palmaz-Schatz Stent

Overall Incidence of Restenosis Following Palmaz-Schatz Stenting

More than 2000 Palmaz-Schatz stents have been placed in native coronary arteries and saphenous vein grafts in the United States and Europe. Sixteen centers have participated in a multicenter registry of this device, contributing both baseline and 6-month angiographic data. A few individual centers have placed large numbers of stents, and have compiled single-center data about restenosis following stenting. Reported angiographic restenosis rates after

Table 2.
Overall Restenosis Rates for Palmaz-Schatz Stents

				Definition of Angiographic		
Ref	*N*	*Vessels*	*Treated*	*Restenosis*	*Follow-up (%)*	*Rate (%)*
Multicenter (early)[36]	247	Native	≥ 50%	?	20	36
Multicenter (core lab)[37]	221	Native	≥ 50%	91	30	37
Beth Israel (1990)[22]	40	RCA	≥ 50%	71	17	
Beth Israel (1992)[18]	250	Native* & SVG	≥ 50%	91	25	
Gutenberg[39]	61	Native & SVG	≥ 50%	84	24	
Toulouse[40]	247	Native	?	83	19	40

SVG = saphenous vein graft, RCA = right coronary artery.
* Single and nontandem multiple stents only.

Palmaz-Schatz stenting have ranged from 17% to 30% using a definition for restenosis of greater than or equal to a 50%–diameter reduction[18,36–40] (Table 2). In the Beth Israel Hospital single-center experience with 250 stent placements, the overall angiographic restenosis rate was 25%, which was lower than expected since 97% of all lesions were associated with one or more factors which traditionally have been associated with an increased predisposition to restenosis.[18] Earlier data from the multicenter and Beth Israel cohorts suggested an even lower rate of restenosis,[36,38] but these initial reports were based on small numbers of patients with predominantly right coronary artery stents. In contrast, more recent data from both sources now include a significant number of stents placed in the native left anterior descending artery and saphenous vein grafts. These overall restenosis rates for the Palmaz-Schatz stent compare favorably to those reported for the Wallstent and Gianturco-Roubin stent.[41,42]

Possible Mechanisms for Decreasing Restenosis

In theory, there are a number of mechanisms by which an endovascular prosthesis might reduce the incidence of restenosis. According to the geometric model of restenosis, these mechanisms can be categorized as those which increase acute gain, and those which decrease late loss. Stenting clearly enhances acute gain by two mechanisms. First, it provides a supporting lattice that allows the operator to safely dilate the vessel with a larger balloon (i.e., a balloon to artery ratio > 1) without increasing the risk of acute closure, as seen when oversized balloons are used for conventional angioplasty.[43] Second, the problems of elastic recoil and vasospasm are largely eliminated in the segment of the artery treated with the Palmaz-Schatz stent. This second mechanism is not present equally for all stents, since the Gianturco-Roubin stent loses approximately 15% to 20% of its expanded diameter due to stent recoil.[41] Finally, stenting may also be associated with decreased late loss. Although this has yet to be demonstrated in humans, Schatz has demonstrated, in human-cadaveric arteries, that the Palmaz-Schatz stent improves flow dynamics, which might reduce the stimulus to smooth muscle cell proliferation.[44]

Patient Factors Associated with Stent Restenosis

Neither age, gender, history of hypertension, hypercholesterolemia, cigarette smoking, recent or remote myocardial infarction, or unstable angina appear to be associated with an increased risk of restenosis following stenting.[18] However, the restenosis rate for patients with diabetes mellitus was significantly greater than for nondiabetics (56% versus 20%; relative risk 2.8).[45] In the multicenter experience, diabetes was also associated with a slight, but not statistically significant, increase in the risk of restenosis.[40] Although several series have documented that diabetes is a predictor of increased risk of restenosis following conventional balloon angioplasty, the pathophysiologic mechanism is uncertain.[46–47]

Lesion Factors Associated with Restenosis

Most investigators believe that the implanted stent should cover the entire lesion. The placement of tandem, overlapping stents was proposed as a way to treat stenoses with lengths exceeding 15 mm. However, the practice of placing tandem stents was soon discontinued due to restenosis rates greater than 50%.[18,39] Multiple stents placed in a single vessel also appear to confer a higher risk of restenosis than single stents.[40] It is uncertain whether the increased incidence of restenosis associated with overlapping stents results from a more exuberant stimulus-to-intimal proliferation in the region of metal overlap, or whether the increased restenosis rate simply reflects the adverse influence of lesion length.[9] The incidence of restenosis following placement of multiple, noncontiguous stents in a single vessel has not been established, but may be intermediate between rates for single and tandem stents.[48] A preliminary report has found that simultaneous or sequential placement of stents in multiple native coronary or saphenous vein grafts confers a similar restenosis risk to single-vessel stenting.[49]

Although the early delivery system for the Palmaz-Schatz stents initially favored right coronary artery placement, availability of a delivery sheath soon led to expansion of the protocol to include placement in the left anterior descending and circumflex arteries, as well as saphenous vein bypass grafts. While the procedural success rate for stenting of the left anterior descending artery appears similar to that of the right coronary artery, the restenosis rate of the left anterior descending is significantly greater than the right coronary artery (44% versus 12%; relative risk 3.67).[18] In the Beth Israel series, the mean-reference artery diameter was slightly, but significantly, smaller for the left anterior descending than for the right coronary artery, but a multivariate analysis that controlled for vessel size showed that stenting of the left anterior descending artery was an independent predictor of restenosis. This finding is in accord with data from the M-HEART study, which showed a similarly greater risk of restenosis in the left anterior descending artery following conventional balloon angioplasty.[9] Ellis found no association between vessel location and rate of restenosis following stenting,[40] but his evaluation was based on a smaller number of stents.

Balloon dilatation of saphenous vein grafts is associated with a risk of restenosis ranging from 40% to 65%.[9,50] Restenosis rates following stent placement in focally diseased vein grafts have been 28% in the multicenter experience,[51] and 25% in the Beth Israel Hospital series.[18] In both series, the restenosis rates for vein grafts were almost identical to those of native coronaries. It is important to note that the multicenter-vein graft cohort had a preponderance of de novo lesions and a larger reference vessel size, factors which tend to be associated with a lower rate of restenosis.

Angioplasty performed in vessels which have been treated previously with balloon dilatation may have a higher incidence of restenosis than de novo lesions.[21,52] In the multicenter experience, Ellis et al found a significantly higher risk of restenosis for previously treated lesions, as compared with de novo lesions (36% versus 16%).[37] Carrozza et al also noted a trend toward higher restenosis rates for previously treated lesions (29% versus 18%), although this difference did not achieve statistical significance.[18] Interestingly, the risk of restenosis following stenting does not appear to be greater in lesions with multiple, rather than a single previous dilatation.[53]

The present generation of Palmaz-Schatz stents may be expanded to a final diameter of between 3 mm and 5 mm. As a result, almost all stents were placed in vessels with diameters exceeding 2.75 mm. Given the lack of experience in stenting smaller arteries, current data for Palmaz-Schatz stents are applicable only to moderate- and large-sized vessels. A recent analysis of conventional angioplasty documents an increased incidence of restenosis in smaller vessels due to an increase in the loss index (late loss/acute gain) for smaller vessels.[54] By a similar analysis, stenting of small arteries might also yield an increased incidence of restenosis, particularly if there is an obligate degree of intimal hyperplasia associated with endothelialization of a stent.

It is unclear whether the morphologic criteria predictive of increased restenosis following balloon angioplasty (e.g., lesion eccentricity, calcification, length, or angulation) also predict increased restenosis following stenting. Analysis of angiographic data from the multicenter-core lab may answer this question. Preliminary data from a small number of patients suggest that stent placement following balloon dilatation of totally occluded coronary arteries is associated with a high (50%) incidence of restenosis.[55] Stenting of ostial stenoses may also result in a slightly higher rate (35%) of restenosis than stents placed in nonostial locations.[56]

Procedure-Related Factors Associated with Restenosis

Palmaz-Schatz stents have been used in three clinical situations: treatment of lesions with a high *a priori* likelihood of restenosis, improvement of suboptimal results following conventional balloon angioplasty, and as a "bailout" device to treat acute vessel closure. Whether the accompanying anatomical and functional differences in the vascular milieu result in differential restenosis rates is unknown. Preliminary data, however, suggest a higher incidence of restenosis when stents are used as a bailout device[41] (see Chapter 6).

A residual stenosis of 20% to 30% is common following conventional angioplasty, and greater residual postprocedure stenosis appears to be a strong predictor of subsequent restenosis.[5,57] Levine has shown that the postprocedure lumen following Palmaz-Schatz stenting is significantly larger than that present after balloon angioplasty.[38] In the Beth Israel Hospital series, a mean-residual stenosis of 0% was observed, and the rate of restenosis was significantly lower in stents with a postprocedure lumen larger than 3.31 mm.[18] In the multicenter experience, a negative residual stenosis (< 0%) was associated with a significantly lower restenosis rate (6% versus 33%).[37] These two findings underscore the concept that restenosis rates following stenting can be reduced by achieving a large posttreatment lumen.

How Does Restenosis Occur Within the Palmaz-Schatz Stent?

Theoretically, stenting may result in a decreased incidence of restenosis compared with conventional balloon angioplasty either by increasing the acute gain, resulting in a smaller residual stenosis, or by decreasing late loss by reducing intimal hyperplasia. The magnitude of acute gain is significantly greater following stenting. Kuntz has shown that the magnitude of late loss following stenting actually *exceeds* that of conventional balloon angioplasty.[24] While related to acute gain, late loss typically is less than half of acute gain, so that a large posttreatment-lumen diameter is the strongest predictor of a large late-lumen diameter.

The quantity of late loss after stenting follows the normal distribution with a mean value of 1.08 mm.[24] Controversy exists as to whether this late loss is explained entirely by ingrowth of intimal hyperplasia, or whether external compression of the stent also contributes to progressive luminal narrowing. Bonner has presented preliminary lumen ultrasound data suggesting that Palmaz-Schatz stents lose approximately 18% of their expanded diameter due to recoil, and are progressively compressed over the next 6 months.[58] However, these measurements are limited by difficulty in differentiating the vascular lumen from the expanded-stent diameter. In our experience, late loss can be explained almost entirely by intimal hyperplasia. This finding is supported by data suggesting that enlargement of the vascular lumen following redilation

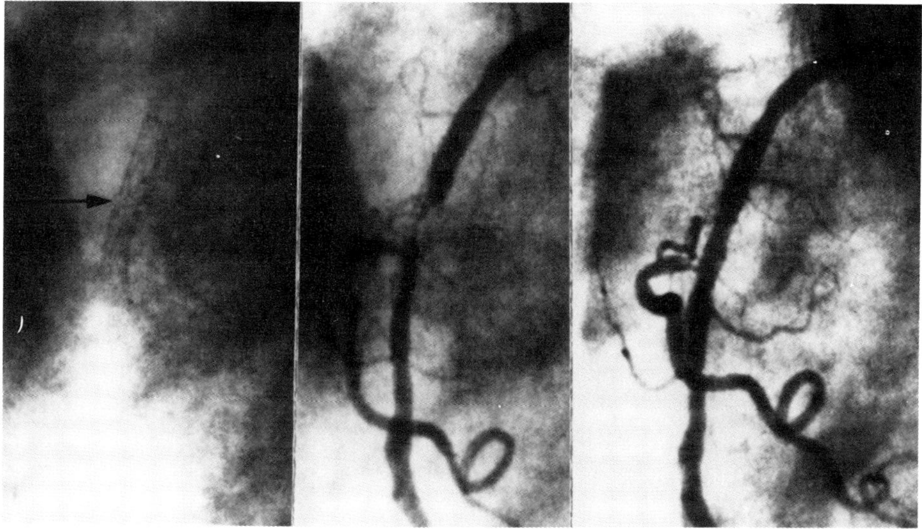

Figure 2: *Restenosis occuring at the articulation site of the Palmaz-Schatz stent. The stent and its articulation site (arrow) is visualized just prior to dye injection (left panel). Focal narrowing is seen at this site when the vessel is opacified (middle panel). Following balloon dilatation within the stent, luminal patency is restored (right panel).*

for in-stent restenosis is due to extrusion of extracellular tissue through the struts of the stent, rather than stent reexpansion.[59]

In a serial angiographic analysis, luminal narrowing following stent placement occurs mostly during the first 3 months, consistent with the known time course of intimal hyperplasia following vascular injury.[60] Beyond 6 months, progressive luminal narrowing is rare.[61] Furthermore, luminal ingrowth of hyperplastic intima does not occur in a homogeneous manner throughout the stent, but appears maximal at the articulation site (Fig. 2).[62] Levine found a mean-neointimal thickening of approximately 500 μg within the stent at 6 months.[38]. In contrast, the mean-intimal thickening within stents placed in normal coronaries of dogs is only approximately 300 μg,[63] and only 270 μ when placed in the coronaries of the atherogenic minipig.[64] This discrepancy in the magnitude of neointimal proliferation might be either species-related, or due to differences in the vascular biology of normal and diseased arteries.

Outcome and Management of In-stent Restenosis

Leon analyzed the clinical outcome of 112 patients with angiographic restenosis.[65] One-third of these patients were asymptomatic and remained free of late clinical events, suggesting that asymptomatic patients with stent restenosis can be managed conservatively. Approximately one-half of patients with restenosis were treated with repeat balloon angioplasty, and 17% with bypass

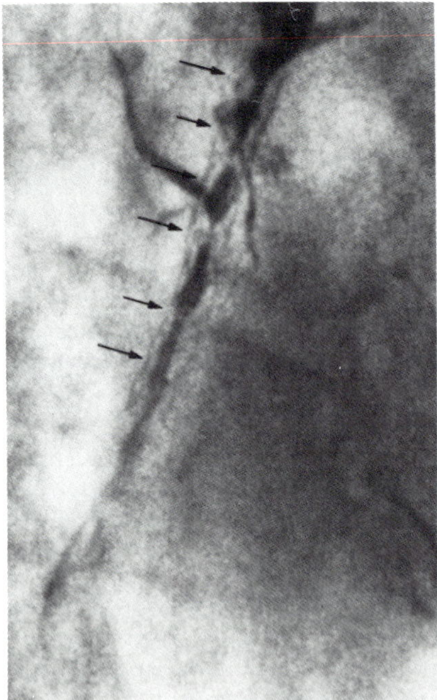
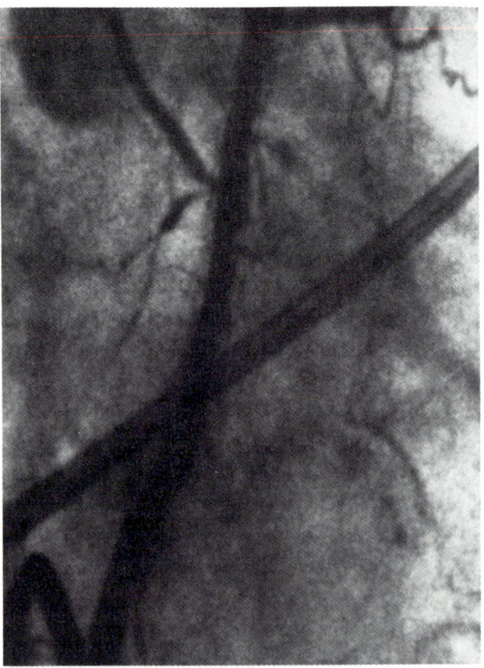

Figure 3: *Successful redilation as treatment for restenosis within tandem Palmaz-Schatz stents. Diffuse luminal narrowing is seen within two contiguous stents (left panel). A smooth lumen is restored following balloon dilatation within both stents (right panel).*

surgery. In the Beth Israel experience, only 12% of patients had a cardiovascular event (death, myocardial infarction, or repeat revascularization) at 6 months, despite a 25% angiographic-restenosis rate.[18] At 3 years, event-free survival remained greater than 70% despite late events unrelated to the stented artery. One-year event-free survival is similar for patients treated with multivessel Palmaz-Schatz stenting.[49]

When in-stent restenosis is associated with objective evidence of myocardial ischemia or angina, repeat balloon dilatation can be safely performed in almost all patients.[66] A near-zero residual stenosis can again be obtained by dilation with a full-sized balloon (Fig. 3). Since the tough neointima does not undergo gross cracking with exposure of stent struts, additional warfarin therapy does not appear necessary. In the multicenter experience, 50% of all patients with in-stent restenosis underwent angioplasty within the stent. The procedure was successful in all patients, without acute closure or embolic events. Follow-up angiography was obtained in 45% of these patients and revealed restenosis in approximately 50% of patients. A "re-re-PTCA" was successfully performed in patients with recurrent restenosis.

Future Directions

At the present time, no large randomized trials comparing restenosis rates after stenting or conventional angioplasty have been completed. The STRESS (Stents in Restenosis Study) trial is a randomized, prospective trial comparing the complication and 6-month restenosis rate of balloon angioplasty and the Palmaz-Schatz stent in discrete, de novo native coronary lesions. A similar trial in Europe (BENESTENT) is also ongoing at this time. These studies will provide a direct comparison of this device with conventional balloon angioplasty using 6-month angiographic restenosis as a primary end point.

Efforts to reduce restenosis have concentrated on two areas: stent design and coating. If the articulation site of the stent does represent a "design flaw" that may provide a locus of luminal ingrowth, future generations of stents with a more subtle articulation may be needed to lower the incidence of restenosis. Dichek has successfully seeded endothelial cells, genetically modified to express the human tissue plasminogen-activator gene onto the struts of stainless-steel stents.[67] In the future, similar techniques might be used to alter expression of smooth muscle cells and decrease the proliferative response accompanying vascular injury.

Conclusions

The Palmaz-Schatz stent is one of several new devices presently under investigation to determine efficacy in reducing restenosis. Until controlled trials such as STRESS are completed, it is difficult to make direct comparisons between the historic restenosis rates following conventional angioplasty and those reported for stents. However, two large series (the multicenter and the single-center Beth Israel experiences) have documented favorable rates of angiographic restenosis when Palmaz-Schatz stents are used to treat discrete lesions in medium- to large-sized arteries. Stenting of diseased saphenous vein grafts appears to have particularly advantageous restenosis rates which may be markedly lower than rates reported for conventional vein graft angioplasty.

The application of a continuous model of restenosis has provided valuable insight into the mechanism by which stents might reduce the incidence of restenosis. Even though stenting does not reduce the magnitude of late loss, it allows safe maximization of the posttreatment-lumen diameter (one of the strongest predictors of restenosis following any coronary intervention).

Despite these encouraging results, restenosis still occurs in 25% of Palmaz-Schatz stents. Predictors of restenosis include stenting of the left anterior descending artery, diabetes mellitus, prior angioplasty, postprocedure-lumen diameter less than 3.30 mm and presence of residual postprocedure stenosis (Table 3). In-stent restenosis can be treated safely by balloon dilatation. Future stent designs and surface modifications may ultimately reduce late loss, and thereby reduce the incidence of restenosis following stenting.

Table 3.
Predictors of Restenosis Following Stenting

	Center	Relative Risk	P[1]
Demographic			
Diabetes mellitus	Beth Israel	2.8	0.006
	Multicenter	1.45	0.14
Angiographic			
Vessel location (LAD)[2]	Beth Israel	3.67	0.002
	Multicenter		>.20
Prior restenosis	Beth Israel	1.47	NS
	Multicenter	2.23	0.04[3]
Reference artery (< 2.5 mm)	Multicenter		0.06
Multiple stents[2]	Multicenter	2.11	0.001
Total occlusion	Multicenter		0.002
Procedural			
Postprocedure lumen diameter < 3.30	Beth Israel	2.12	0.05
Postprocedure stenosis > 0%	Multicenter		0.05

[1] Univariable analysis
[2] Independent predictor by multivariable analysis
[3] Single stents only

REFERENCES

1. Gruentzig, AR, Senning A, Siegenthaler WE: Nonoperative dilatation of coronary artery stenosis-percutaneous transluminal angioplasty. *N Engl J Med* 1979; 301: 61–68.
2. Holmes DR, Vliestra RE, Smith HC, Vetrovec G, Kent KM, Cowley MJ, Faxon DP, Gruentzig AR, Kelsey SF, Detre KM, van Raden MJ, Mock MB: Restenosis after percutaneous transluminal coronary angioplasty (PTCA): a report from the PTCA Registry of the National Heart, Lung, and Blood Institute. *Am J Cardiol* 1984; 53: 77C-81C.
3. Detre K, Holubkov R, Kelsey S, Cowley MJ, Kent K, Williams D, Myler R, Faxon D, Holmes D Jr, Bourassa M, Block P, Gosselin A, Bentivoglio L, Leatherman L, Dorros G, King S, Galichia J, Al-Bassam M, Leon M, Robertson T, Passamani E, and the coinvestigators of the National Heart, Lung, and Blood Institute's Percutaneous Transluminal Coronary Angioplasty Registry: Percutaneous transluminal coronary angioplasty in 1985–1986 and 1977–1981. *N Engl J Med* 1988; 318:265–270.
4. Gruentzig AR, King SB III, Schlumpf M, Siegenthaler W: Long-term follow-up after percutaneous transluminal coronary angioplasty: the early Zurich experience. *N Engl J Med* 1987; 316:1127–1132.
5. Guiteras V, Bourassa MG, David PR, Bonan R, Crepeau J, Dyrda I, Lesperance J: Restenosis after successful percutaneous coronary angioplasty: The Montreal Heart Institute experience. *Am J Coll Cardiol* 1987; 60:50B-55B.
6. Kaltenbach M, Kober G, Scherer D, Vallbracht C: Recurrence after successful coronary angioplasty. *Eur Heart J* 1985; 6:276–281.
7. Serruys PW, Luijten HE, Beatt R, Geuskens BR, DeFeyter PJ, van den Brand M, Reiber JHC, Ten Kate HJ, van Es GA, Hugenholtz PG: Incidence of restenosis

after successful coronary angioplasty: a time-related phenomenon. A quantitative angiographic study in 342 consecutive patients at 1,2,3 and 4 months. *Circulation* 1988; 77:361–371.

8. Nobuyoshi M, Kimura T, Nosaka H, Mioka S, Ueno K, Yokoi H, Hamasaki N, Horiuchi H, Ohishi H: Restenosis after successful percutneous transluminal coronary angioplasty: serial angiographic follow-up of 229 patients. *J Am Coll Cardiol* 1988; 12:616–623.
9. Hirshfeld JW, Schwartz JS, Jugo R, Macdonald RG, Goldberg S, Savage MP, Bass TA, Vetrovec G, Cowley M, Taussig AS, Whitworth HB, Margolis JR, Hill JA, Pepine CJ and the M-HEART Investigators: Restenosis after coronary angioplasty: a multivariate statistical model to relate lesion and procedure variables to restenosis. *J Am Coll Cardiol* 1991; 18:647–656.
10. Thornton MA, Gruentzig AR, Hollman J, King SB III, Douglas JS Jr: Coumadin and aspirin in prevention of recurrence after transluminal coronary angioplasty: a randomized study. *Circulation* 1984; 69:721–727.
11. Ellis SG, Roubin GS, Wilentz J, Douglas JS, King SB III: Effects of 18–24 hours of heparin administration for prevention of restenosis after uncomplicated coronaryangioplasty. *Am Heart J* 1989; 117:777–782.
12. Corcos T, David PR, Val PG, Renken J, Dangoisse V, Rapold HG, Bourassa MG: Failure of diltiazam to prevent restenosis after percutaneous transluminal coronary angioplasty. *Am Heart J* 1985; 109:926–931.
13. Grigg LE, Kay TWH, Valentine PA: Determinants of restenosis and lack of effect of dietary supplementation with eicosopentaenoic acid on the incidence of coronary artery restenosis after angioplasty. *J Am Coll Cardiol* 1989; 13:665–672.
14. Pepine CJ, Hirshfeld JW, Macdonald RG, Henderson MA, Bass TA, Goldberg S, Savage MP, Vetrovec G, Cowley M, Taussig AS, Whitworth HE, Margolis JR, Hill JA, Bove AA, Jugo R: A controlled trial of corticosteroids to prevent restenosis following coronary angioplasty. *Circulation* 1990; 81:1753–1761.
15. Spears JR, Reyes VP, Wynne J, Fromm BS, Sikofsky EL, Andrus S, et al: Percutaneous coronary laser balloon angioplasty: initial results of a multicenter experience. *J Am Col Cardiol* 1990; 16:293–303.
16. Fishman RF, Kuntz RE, Carrozza JP, Miller MJ, Senerchia CC, Schnitt SJ, Diver DJ, Safian L, Baim DS: Long-term results of directional coronary atherectomy: Predictors of restenosis. *J Am Coll Cardiol* 1992;20:1101–1110.
17. Serruys PW, Strauss BH, Beatt KJ, Bertrand ME, Puel J, Rickards AF, Meier B, Goy JJ, Vogt P, Kappenberger L, Sigwart U: Angiographic follow-up after placement of a self-expanding coronary-artery stent. *N Engl J Med* 1991; 324:13–17.
18. Carrozza JP Jr, Kuntz RE, Levine MJ, et al: Angiographic and clinical outcome of intracoronary stenting: acute and long-term results from a large single-center experience. *J Am Coll Cardiol* (in press).
19. Brozovich FV, Morganroth J, Gottlieb NB, Gottlieb RS: Effect of angiotensin converting enzyme inhibition on the incidence of restenosis after percutaneous transluminal coronary angioplasty. *Cathet Cardiovasc Diagn* 1991; 23:263–267.
20. Leimgruber PP, Roubin GS, Hollman J, Cotsonis GA, Meier B, Douglas JS, King SB, Greuntzig, AR: Restenosis after successful coronary angioplasty in patients with single vessel disease. *Circulation* 1986; 73:710–717.
21. Califf RM, Ohman EM, Frid DJ, Fortin DF, Mark, DB, Hlatky MA, Herndon JE, Bengtson JR: Restenosis: the clinical issues. In: Topol E, ed. *Textbook of Interventional Cardiology*. Philadephia: WB Saunders & Co, Inc; 1990, 363–394.
22. Levine MJ, Baim DS, Schatz RA, Fischman DL, Hirshfeld JW: Subpopulation differences in restenosis after coronary stenting: a definition-independent evaluation. *Circlation* 1990 (suppl III):656a. Abstract.
23. Forrester JS, Fishbein M, Helfant R, Fagin J: A paradigm for restenosis based on cell biology: clues for the development of new preventative therapies. *J Am Coll Cardiol* 1991; 17:758–769.

24. Kuntz RE, Safian RD, Levine MJ, Reis GS, Diver DJ, Baim DS: A novel approach to the analysis of restenosis following three new coronary devices. *J Am Coll Cardiol* 1992; 19:1493–1499.
25. Bobbio M, Detrano R, Colombo A, Lehmann KG, Park JB: Restenosis rate after percutaneous transluminal coronary angioplasty: a literature overview. *J Invasive Cardiol* 1991; 3:214–224.
26. Ernst SMPG, van den Feltz TA, Bal ET, Bogerijen LV, Van Den Berg E, Ascoop CAPL, Plokker HM: Long-term angiographic follow-up, cardiac events, and survival in patients undergoing percutaneous transluminal coronary angioplasty. *Br Heart J* 1987; 57:220–225.
27. Lambert M, Bonan R, Cote G, Crepeau J, de Geuse P, Lesperance J, David PR, Walters DD: Multiple coronary angioplasty: a model to discriminate systemic and procedural factors related to restenosis. *J Am Coll Cardiol* 1988; 12:310–314.
28. Meier B: Total coronary occlusion: a different animal? *J Am Coll Cardiol* 1991; 17: 50B-57B.
29. Ellis SG, Roubin GS, King SB III, Douglas JS Jr, Cox WR: Importance of stenosis morphology in the estimation of restenosis risk after elective percutaneous transluminal coronary angioplasty. *Am J Cardiol* 1989; 63:30–34.
30. Waller BF, Pinkerton CA, Orr CM, Stack JD, Van Tossel JW, Peters T: Restenosis 1–24 months after successful balloon angioplasty: A necropsy study of 20 patients. *J Am Coll Cardiol* 1991; 17:58B-70B.
31. Uchida Y, Hosegawa K, Kawamura K, Shibuya I: Angioscopic observation of coronary angioplasty. *Am Heart J* 1989; 117:769–776.
32. Safian RD, Gelbfish JS, Erny RE, Schnitt SJ, Schmidt DA, Baim DS: Coronary atherectomy: clinical, angiographic and histologic findings and observations regarding potential mechanisms *Circulation* 1990; 82:69–79.
33. Muller DWM, Ellis SG, Topol EJ: Experimental models of coronary restenosis. *J Am Coll Cardiol* 1992; 19:418–432.
34. Rensing BJ, Hermans WR, Strauss BH, Serruys PW: Regional differences in elastic recoil after percutaneous transluminal coronary angioplasty: a quantitative angiographic study. *J Am Coll Cardiol* 1991; 17:34B-38B.
35. Fischell TA, Derby G, Tse TM, Stadius ML: Coronary artery vasoconstriction routinely occurs after percutaneous transluminal coronary angioplasty: a quantitative arteriographic analysis *Circulation* 1988; 78:1323–1334.
36. Schatz RA, Goldberg S, Leon M, Baim D, Hirshfeld JW, Cleman M, Ellis S, Topol E: Clinical experience with the Palmaz-Schatz coronary stent. *J Am Coll Cardiol* 1991; 17:155B-159B.
37. Ellis SG, Savage M, Fischman D, Baim DS, Leon M, Goldberg S, Hirshfeld JW, Cleman MW, Tierstein PS, Walker C, Bailey S, Buchbinder M, Topol EJ, Schatz RA: Restenosis after placement of Palmaz-Schatz stents in native coronary arteries: initial results of a multicenter experience. *Circulation* 1992; 86:1836–1844.
38. Levine MJ, Leonard BM, Burke JA, Nash ID, Safian RD, Diver DJ, Baim DS: Clinical and angiographic results of balloon expandable intracoronary stents in right coronary artery stenoses. *J Am Coll Cardiol* 1990; 16: 332–339.
39. Haude M, Erbel R, Straube U, Dietz U, Meyer J: Short- and long-term results after intracoronary stenting in human coronary arteries: monocentre experience with balloon-expandable Palmaz-Schatz stent. *Br Heart J* 1991; 66:337–345.
40. Fajadet J, Jenny D, Guagliumi G, Cassagneau B, Robert G, Marco J: Does the indication for coronary stenting influence clinical results? *J Am Coll Cardiol* 1992; 19:198A. Abstract.
41. Roubin GS, Adam CD, Agrawal SK, Macander PJ, Dean LS, Baxley WA, Breland J: Intracoronary stenting for acute and threatened closure complicating percutaneous transluminal coronary angioplasty. *Circulation* 1992; 85:916–927.
42. Strauss BH, Serruys PW, de Scheerder IK, Tijssen JGP, Bertrand ME, Puel J, Meier B, Kaufmann U, Stauffer JC, Rickards AE, Sigwart U: Relative risk of angiographic

predictors for restenosis within the coronary Wallstent. *Circulation* 1991; 84: 1636–1644.

43. Roubin GS, Douglas JS, King SB, Lin S, Hutchison N, Thomas RG, Gruentzig AR: Influence of balloon size on initial success, acute complications and restenosis after percutaneous transluminal coronary angioplasty: a prospective, randomized study. *Circulation* 1988; 78:557–565.
44. Schatz RA: A view of vascular stents. *Circulation* 1989; 79:445–457.
45. Carrozza JP, Kuntz RE, Fishman RF, Baim DS: Restenosis following arterial injury in diabetics: an analysis of intimal hyperplasia following coronary stenting. *Ann Intern Med* 1993;118:344–349.
46. Quigley PJ, Hlatky MA, Hinohara T, Randall DS, Perez JA, Phillips HR, Califf RM, Stack RS: Repeat percutaneous transluminal coronary angioplasty and predictors of recurrent restenosis. *Am J Cardiol* 1989; 63:409–413.
47. Myler RK, Topol EJ, Shaw RE, Stertzer SH, Clark DA, Fishman J, Murphy MC: Multiple vessel coronary angioplasty: classification, results, and patterns of restenosis in 494 consecutive patients. *Cathet Cardiovasc Diagn* 1987; 13:1–15.
48. Buchbinder M, Reisman M, Fischman D, Savage M, Bailey SR: Outcome in patients treated with multiple stent implants in a single vessel. *J Am Coll Cardiol* 1992; 19:11OA. Abstract.
49. Carrozza JP, Kuntz RE, Fishman RF, Friedrich S, Miller MJ, Baim DS: Multivessel Palmaz-Schatz stenting. *Coronary Artery Disease* 1993 (in press).
50. Cote G, Myler RK, Stertzer SH, Clark DA, Fishman-Rosen J, Murphy M, Straw RE: Percutaneous transluminal angioplasty of stenotic coronary artery bypass grafts: 5 years' experience. *J Am Coll Cardiol* 1987; 9:8–17.
51. Leon MB, Kent KM, Baim DS, Walker CM, Cleman MW, Buchbinder M, Heuser FF, Curry C, Schatz, RA: Comparison of stent implantation in native coronaries and saphenous vein grafts. *J Am Coll Cardiol* 1992; 19:263A. Abstract.
52. Teirstein PS, Hoover C, Ligon B, Giorgi LV, Rutherford BD, McConahay DR, Johnson WL, Hartzler GO: Repeat restenosis: efficacy of the third and fourth coronary angioplasty *J Am Coll Cardiol* 1987; 9:63A. Abstract.
53. Savage M, Fischman D, Leon M, Ellis S, Schatz R, Goldberg S: Restenosis risk of single Palmaz-Schatz stents in native coronaries: report from the core angiographic laboratory. *J Am Coll Cardiol* 1992; 19:277A. Abstract.
54. Kuntz RE, Nobuyoshi M, Gibson CM, Baim DS: Generalized model of restenosis following conventional balloon angioplasty, stenting and directional atherectomy. *J Am Coll Cardiol* 1993;21:15–25.
55. Cleman MW, Calim HS, Schatz RA, Goldberg S, Walker C: Intracoronary stenting after PTCA of totally occluded arteries. *Circulation* 1989; (suppl II):258A. Abstract.
56. Teirstein P, Stratienko AA, Schatz RA: Coronary stenting for ostial stenoses: initial results and 6-month follow-up.*Circulation* 1991; (suppl II) 84:250a. Abstract.
57. Lambert M, Bonan R, Cote G, Crepeau J, de Guise P, Lesperance J, David PR, Waters DD: Multiple coronary angioplasty: a model to discriminate systemic and procedural factors related to restenosis. *J Am Coll Cardiol* 1988; 12:310–314.
58. Bonner RF, Karen G, Douek PC, Leon MB: Acute and chronic compression of rigid slotted stents account for progressive lumen narrowing. *Circulation* 1991; (suppl II) 84:197A. Abstract.
59. Macdonald RG, O'Neill BJ, Creighton JE, Brown RI, Silvocka JE, Penn IM: Is coronary stent expansion the mechanism for successful dilatation of stent restenosis? A quantitative angiographic follow-up. *Circulation* 1991; (suppl:II) 84:196A. Abstract.
60. Kimura T, Nobuyoshi M, Nosaka H, Yokoi H, Hamasaki N: Palmaz-Schatz balloon-expandable coronary stent: serial angiographic follow-up. *Circulation* 1991; (suppl II) 84:589A. Abstract.
61. Savage M, Fischman D, Ellis S, Leon M, Cleman M, Teirstein PS, Walker C, Hirshfeld J, Schatz RA, Goldberg S: Does late progression of restenosis occur beyond 6

months following coronary artery stenting? *Circulation* 1990; (suppl III); 82:540A. Abstract.
62. Penn IM, Galligan L, Brown RI, Murray-Parsons N, Foley JB, White J: Restenosis at the stent articulation: is this a design flaw? *J Am Coll Cardiol* 1992; 19:291A. Abstract.
63. Schatz RA, Palmaz JC, Tio FO, Garcia F, Garcia 0, Reuter SR: Balloon-expandable intracoronary stents in the adult dog. *Circulation* 1987; 76:450–457.
64. White CJ, Ramee SR, Banks AK, Mesa JE, Chokshi S, Isner JM: A new balloon-expandable tantalum coil stent: angiographic patency and histologic findings in an atherogenic swine model. *J Am Coll Cardiol* 1992; 19:870–876.
65. Leon MB, Baim DS, Goldberg S, Teirstein PS, Hirshfeld JW, Ellis SG, Pichard AD, Schatz RA: Long-term angiographic and clinical follow-up after placement of coronary stents. *J Am Coll Cardiol* 1992; 19:197A. Abstract.
66. Baim DS, Levine MJ, Leon M, Teirstein P, Schatz RA and the U.S. Palmaz-Schatz Stent Investigators: Management of restenosis within Palmaz-Schatz intracoronary stents: multicenter results. *Am J Cardiol* 1993;71:364–366.
67. Dichek DA, Neville RF, Zweibel JA, Freeman SM, Leon MB, Anderson WF: Seeding of intravascular stents with genetically engineered endothelial cells. *Circulation* 1989; 80:1347–1353.

CHAPTER 6

Emergent Stenting for Failed Percutaneous Transluminal Coronary Angioplasty

Howard C. Herrmann
John W. Hirshfeld, Jr.

During the last decade, percutaneous transluminal coronary angioplasty (PTCA) has become the most frequently used coronary revascularization procedure in the United States with more than 300,000 procedures performed annually. Success rates generally exceed 90%, despite the rapid expansion into new indications including unstable angina, acute myocardial infarction, more complex lesions, and multivessel diseases.[1] However, PTCA is still limited by a disturbingly high rate of restenosis (30% to 45%), inability to cross or dilate some lesions (5% to 10%), and abrupt vessel occlusion during or shortly after the procedure (2% to 9%). The Palmaz-Schatz balloon-expandable stent was developed to address some of these problems. This chapter will address the emergent use of the Palmaz-Schatz stent for acute and impending vessel closure after PTCA.

Acute Occlusion: Incidence and Mechanisms

Acute occlusion occurring during or within 24 hours of PTCA occurs in only a minority of procedures, but is associated with a high rate of serious complications.[2–11]

Examination of Table 1, which lists most reported studies of acute occlusion, reveals that the mean incidence of this complication in 806 reported cases of patients undergoing angioplasty is 6.1% (range 2.0% to 8.5%). A similar rate of acute occlusion has been reported in patients undergoing multilesion angioplasty, but these patients may experience an even higher rate of complications.[12] Differences in the reported rates are due to differences in the definition

From: Herrmann HC, Hirshfeld JW, eds. *Clinical Use of the Palmaz-Schatz Intracoronary Stent.* Futura Publishing Company, Inc., Mount Kisco, NY, © 1993.

Table 1.
Reported Series of Acute and Impending Closure ≤24h after PTCA

Reference	N	Incidence	Complications: Death	CABG	Total MI (Q-Wave Only)
Cowley, 1984[2]	151	4.9%	5%	72%	41%
Shiu, 1985[3]	20	8.3%	10%	65%	25%
Simpfendorfer, 1987[4]	32	2.0%	0	41%	(43%)
Ellis, 1988[5]	140	4.4%	3%	55%	81% (40%)
Meyerovitz, 1988[6]	44	8.5%	2%	30%	
Sinclair, 1988[7]	54	4.7%	2%	22%	35%
Steffenino, 1988[8]	30	6.8%	0	27%	50%
Detre, 1990[9]	122	6.8%	5%	40%	40%
DeFeyter, 1991[10]	104	7.3%	6%	30%	36%
Lincoff, 1992[11]	109	8.3%	8%	20%	20% (9%)
Weighted means:	806	6.1%	4.6%	43%	50% (33%)

PTCA: percutaneous transluminal coronary angioplasty; CABG = coronary artery bypass graft; MI = myocardial infarction.

of acute occlusion (some studies have included threatened closure), inclusion of patients presenting with acute myocardial infarction in some studies, variable study intervals after PTCA up to 24 hours, different time lengths of angiographic observation after the final balloon inflation, and differences in treatment techniques for suboptimal results preceding total occlusion.

In most cases, the mechanism of abrupt closure appears to involve a combination of thrombus formation, creation of tissue flaps due to intimal dissection, and luminal narrowing due to elastic recoil and vascular spasm.[11] The precise cause in a specific patient can only be inferred from the angiographic appearance of the vessel just before occlusion. Thrombus often appears as rounded luminal-filling defects with contrast agent on three sides, may be mobile, and gradually expands to fill the lumen.[13] Intimal dissection is characterized by a filling defect with extraluminal extravasation and/or persistent staining of dye.[13] Neither of these angiographic definitions has been well validated. Furthermore, in practice, thrombus and dissection often occur together, making an exact determination of the cause of vessel occlusion difficult.

Several investigators have examined the preprocedural angiographic factors which are associated with acute occlusion after angioplasty. Factors that have been identified include complex lesion morphology with irregular borders, intraluminal filling defects, the appearance of intimal dissection, eccentric lesions, long lesions, and lesions on a bend.[4,5,9,14–17] However, once the vessel occludes, the exact mechanism responsible for occlusion may not be readily identifiable. In this regard, some of the newer imaging modalities such as angioscopy or intravascular ultrasound may prove useful. Both techniques can directly image dissection flaps and intraluminal thrombus.[18] Angioplasty balloons and devices which incorporate intravascular ultrasound transducers are undergoing evaluation, and may be particularly helpful in elucidating the cause of an abrupt occlusion during the procedure.[19]

As shown in Table 1, acute occlusion after PTCA is associated with a high rate of complications. As many as half of these patients will require emergent bypass surgery, and a similar proportion will suffer a Q- or non-Q-wave myocardial infarction (MI). Furthermore, in studies of emergent coronary artery bypass graft (CABG) after failed PTCA, the incidence of perioperative Q-wave MI (21% to 39%) and death (1.4% to 6.8%) was several times higher than in comparable patient populations undergoing elective surgery.[20–23] Overall, acute occlusion may result in a 5% incidence of death, and accounts for the majority of PTCA-associated mortality[24] (Table 1).

Interventions that have been employed to salvage failed PTCA have included: repeat balloon inflations, administration of intracoronary thrombolytic agents such as urokinase, prolonged balloon inflations with an autoperfusion balloon, laser-balloon angioplasty, stents, and atherectomy. Table 2 summarizes the results of several reported series with these interventions, which are also discussed below. Unfortunately, the lack of uniform patient selection, different criteria for using the chosen intervention, and various definitions for success make direct comparison of success rates with these modalities difficult.

Table 2.
Interventions Used to Salvage Failed PTCA

Intervention	*Reference*	*N*	*Success Rates: Initial (Final)*	*Definitions of Success: Initial (Final)*
1. Intracoronary thrombolysis:	Vaitkus[13]	27	37% (52%)	2 (3)
	Schieman[25]	48	90% (98%)	2 (3)
	Gulba[26]	27	82% (42%)	1 (3)
2. Prolonged balloon inflations (including autoperfusion balloons):	Saenz[27]	22	100% (68%)	1 (3)
	Leitschuh[28]	22	86% (55%)	2 (3)
	Lincoff[11]	37	— (48%)	—(3)
	Vaitkus[13]	17	71% (76%)	2 (3)
3. Laser-balloon angioplasty:	Ferguson[29]	21	95% (86%)	1 (5)
4. Atherectomy:	Whitlow[30]	30	87% (83%)	1 (5)
5. Stents				
Palmaz-Schatz	Herrmann[31]	56	98% (71%)	1 (4)
	Haude[32]	15	100% (87%)	1 (4)
Gianturo-Roubin	Roubin[33]	119	93% (74%)	1 (3)
Wallstent	Sigwart[34]	11	100% (82%)	1 (3)
	deFeyter[35]	15	87% (73%)	1 (3)

Definitions: 1 = open artery; 2 = <50% final stenosis; 3 = freedom in hospital; MI/CABG/death; 4 = 30-day freedom; MI/CABG/death; 5 = 30 day freedom; death & CABG only. MI = myocardial infarction; CABG = coronary artery bypass graft.

Results of Emergent Stenting

Although the balloon-expandable intracoronary stent of Palmaz and Schatz was originally introduced for use in anatomical situations considered unfavorable for conventional balloon angioplasty and for the prevention of restenosis (see Chapters 1, 4, and 5), its mechanism of action would suggest that it might also be effective in salvaging certain PTCA failures. In the setting of luminal obstruction due to a dissection flap, stenting may seal the dissection flap against the vascular wall. This action may protect against further propagation of the dissection as well as reducing vascular occlusion by the flap. In the setting of elastic recoil, the implanted stent may provide a force which permanently opposes this tendency. In both cases, the stent may rapidly reestablish flow to allow the administration of intracoronary pharmacologic agents and abort ischemia.

In order to assess the usefulness of stenting for failed PTCA, we performed a retrospective study examining the results of emergent unplanned coronary artery stenting in United States centers using the Palmaz-Schatz stent. A total of 56 patients received emergentstents in a nonprotocol fashion at seven centers over a 2 and 1/2-year period. The medical records and angiograms of these patients were reviewed to determine the reason for stenting, the results, complications, predictors of outcome, and restenosis rates.[31]

Baseline characteristics of the study population included a mean (± SD) age of 58 ± 11 years and a large prevalence of angiographic characteristics generally considered unfavorable for PTCA including lesion eccentricity (49%), intimal dissection (9%), or angiographically-visible thrombus (6%). Thirty-one percent of patients had undergone a prior angioplasty of the target lesion, and 51% had experienced unstable angina at rest before the planned procedure. The reasons for stent implantation included a suboptimal angiographic result considered unacceptable by the individual investigator in 23 patients (41%), impending closure after PTCA defined as a decrease of greater than or equal to a 1 thrombolysis in myocardial infarction (TIMI) flow grade, with clinical evidence of ischemia including chest pain and electrocardiographic (ECG) changes in 15 patients (27%), and acute occlusion following PTCA defined as TIMI-flow grade 0 or 1, and greater than or equal to a 99% stenosis in 18 patients (32%).

Angiographic characteristics of the postangioplasty (prestent) lesions revealed an increased incidence of intimal dissection (74%), thrombus formation (38%), or both (28%) compared to the baseline angiogram preangioplasty (all $P < 0.05$); only 17% of patients had neither dissection nor thrombus postangiography (Fig. 1). The overall mean stenosis severity postangioplasty was unchanged from preangioplasty (70 ± 27%), and was highest in the patients with impending closure (74 ± 12%) and acute occlusion (99 ± 4%) (Fig. 2).

Grouping only the patients with impending and acute occlusion together, successful stent deployment was achieved in 32/33 patients (96%). Two stents were placed for guide catheter-induced dissections, and the remainder were deployed at the site of the original angioplasty lesion. Examples of successful

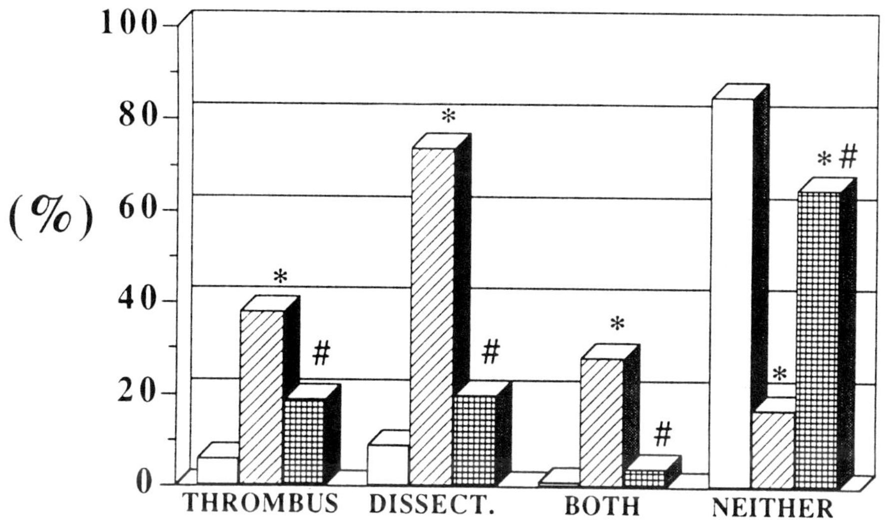

Figure 1: *Angiographic lesion characteristics in 56 patients preangioplasty (open bars), after conventional balloon angioplasty (hatched bars), and after emergency stent implantation (cross-hatched bars); *P* < 0.05 versus pre; *#P* < 0.05 versus post. Note the increased incidence of thrombus and dissection after angioplasty, and the improvement with stenting. (From,[25] with permission).

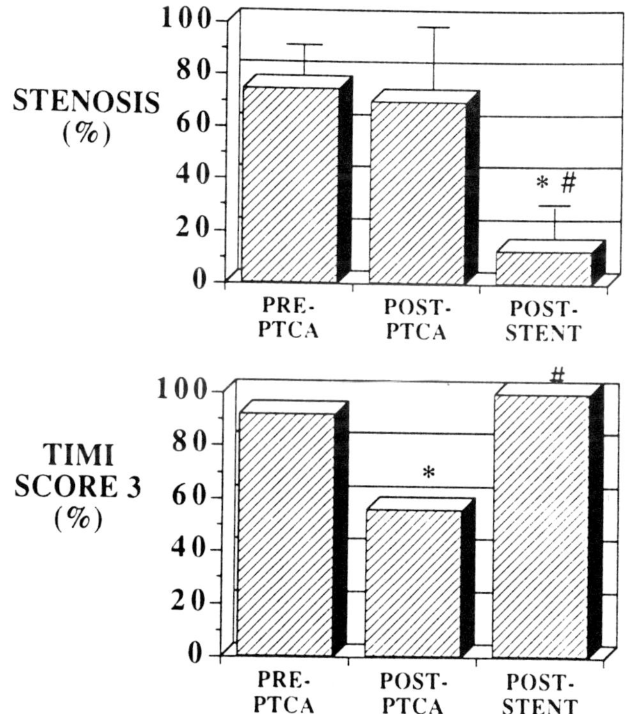

Figure 2: *The percentage stenosis (upper panel) and percentage of patients with a TIMI perfusion score of 3 (lower panel) before PTCA, after PTCA, and after emergent stenting; *P* < 0.05 versus pre-PTCA, *#P* < 0.05 versus post-PTCA. (From,[25] with permission).

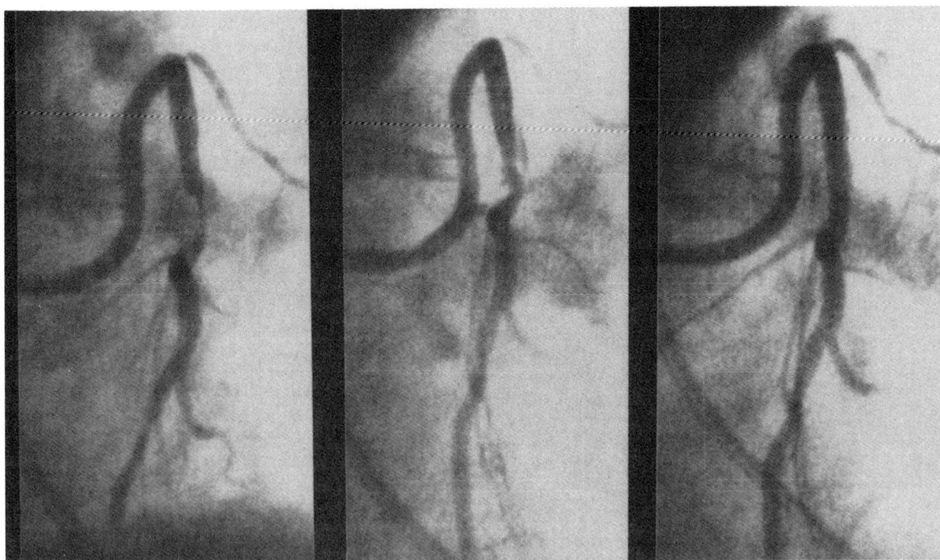

Figure 3: *Angiographic example of emergent unplanned coronary artery stenting to salvage a failed angioplasty with impending vessel closure. The patient developed an intimal dissection which was associated with progressive vessel obstruction and ischemia (middle panel). The dissection was successfully sealed by a stent (right panel).*

stent deployments are shown for impending closure due to a large dissection (Fig. 3), acute occlusion due to both dissection and thrombus (Fig. 4), and acute occlusion following a guide-dissection Fig. 5). Following stent implantation, thrombus and dissection were present in 19% and 20%, respectively, of all angiograms and the mean-percentage stenosis decreased to 13 ± 12% (Fig. 1 and 2).

Initial success (freedom from MI, CABG, and death) was achieved in 31/33 (94%) of the patients with impending and acute occlusion. However, the success rate at 1 month fell to 70% due primarily to the occurrence of subacute stent thrombosis (18%) and its associated complications (Table 3). Major complications occurred in 44% of the acute occlusion subgroup and 13% of patients with impending closure, and could not be predicted by any of 20 variables studied by logistic-regression analysis. Minor complications included groin (14%) and hemorrhagic (13%) problems.

Nine patients, 16% of the entire study population, suffered subacute thromboses at a mean of 5 ± 3 days (range 1 to 10 days) after stent implantation. This occurred despite therapeutic anticoagulation in five of the patients, and all suffered a major complication. Table 4 shows a comparison of parameters in patients with and without subacute thrombosis. The only factor that predicted subacute thrombosis in logistic-regression analysis was the presence

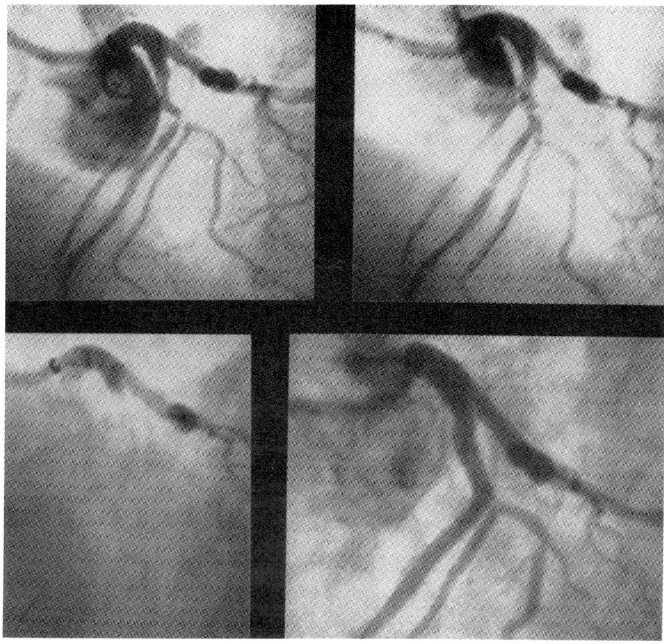

Figure 4: *Angiograms demonstrating salvage of an acute occlusion with a stent. The initial lesion (upper left panel) is a complex bifurcation lesion involving the left anterior descending and diagonal branch arteries. Double-wire balloon angioplasty was complicated by the development of intimal dissection and intraluminal thrombus (upper right panel). Vessel occlusion occurred (lower left panel) despite multiple balloon inflations and intracoronary urokinase administration. Flow was reestablished after stent implantation (lower right). (From,[25] with permission).*

of angiographically-visible thrombus poststent implantation as shown in Figure 6.

During 6 months of follow-up, five patients died; stent thrombosis could have occurred in one of these patients. Excluding patients who died, had subacute thrombosis, or underwent bypass surgery, 85% of eligible patients underwent planned angiography 6 months after stenting. Restenosis (> 50%–diameter reduction) was present in 23% of patients.

Several preliminary investigations have also examined the outcome of emergent Palmaz-Schatz coronary stenting after failed PTCA. In these studies from Germany,[24] Japan,[36] France,[37] Canada,[38] and the Netherlands,[39] a total of 265 patients received emergent Palmaz-Schatz stents. Initial vessel stabilization was achieved in a high proportion of cases (89% to 100%), but major complications including subacute thrombosis were common (13% to 51%). Haude examined the emergent use of this device in 15 patients with coronary dissection and ischemia after balloon angioplasty, similar to the impending-closure group we described above. Although initial successful salvage was

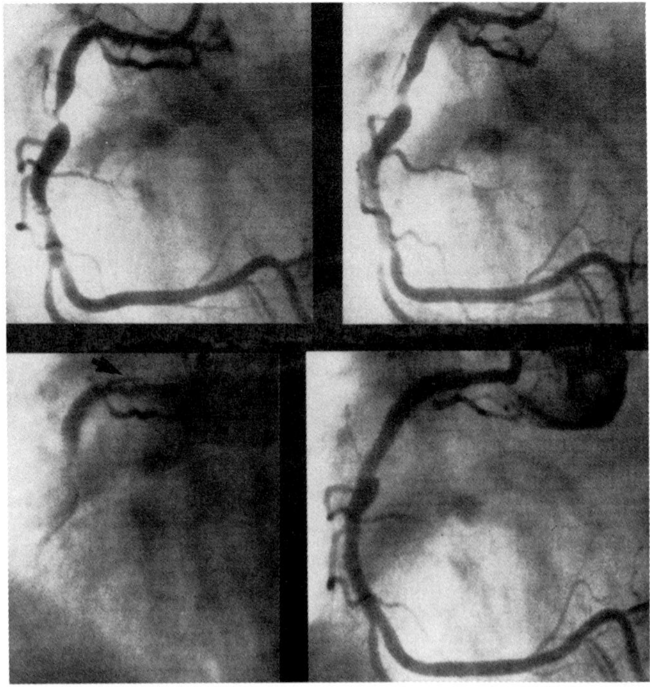

Figure 5: *Example of a patient who underwent angioplasty of an eccentric mid-right coronary artery stenosis (upper right panel) and developed a spiral dissection induced by the guide catheter (arrow), resulting in acute vessel occlusion (lower left panel). Two stents were implanted from just distal to the original stenosis back to near the origin of the vessel. Follow-up angiography 4 months later demonstrated excellent flow with only a small residual dissection (lower right panel).*

Table 3.
Major complications by Subgroup

	MI (Q- & non-Q)	*CABG*	*Death*	*SAT*	*Patients*
Suboptimal result	4	2	1	3	6/23 (26%)
Impending closure	0	1	1	0	2/15 (13%)
Acute occlusion	7	4	0	6	8/18 (44%)
Total (%)	11 (20%)	7 (13%)	2 (4%)	9 (16%)	16/56 (29%)

CABG = Coronary artery bypass graft; MI = myocardial infarction (Q- and non-Q-wave); SAT = subacute thrombosis.

Table 4.
Comparison of Parameters in Patients With and Without Subacute Thrombosis

Parameter	*Subacute Thrombosis*	*No Subacute Thrombosis*	*P**
Baseline Characteristics			
1. Patients (N)	16%	84%	—
2. Age (years)	55 ± 12	58 ± 11	NS
3. Sex (% male)	78%	74%	NS
4. Prior PTCA (%)	33%	30%	NS
5. Unstable angina (%)	22%	51%	NS
Prestent Angiographic Factors			
6. Eccentricity (%)	56%	48%	NS
7. ACC Class (% B)	100%	66%	0.01
8. Thrombus post-PTCA (%)	56%	34%	NS
9. Dissection post-PTCA (%)	67%	75%	NS
10. Acute occlusion subgroup (%)	67%	26%	0.03
Stent-Related Factors			
11. Final stent balloon size (mm)	3.2 ± 2.5	3.4 ± 4.6	NS
12. Multiple stents (%)	22%	20%	NS
13. Poststent residual stneosis (%)	21 ± 13%	12 ± 12%	0.04
14. Thrombus poststent	44%	13%	0.03#
15. Dissection poststent	0%	24%	NS

* Univariate comparisons (NS = $P > 0.05$).
# $P < 0.05$ in multiple stepwise logistic regression analysis.
PTCA: percutaneous transluminal coronary angioplasty.

achieved in all patients, major complications occurred in 27%.[32] Other stents which have been used to salvage failed angioplasty procedures include the Wallstent (Medinvent, Inc., Switzerland) and Gianturco-Roubin stent (Cook, Inc., Bloomington, IN). The Wallstent has a self-expanding mesh design and was implanted in 11 patients with acute vessel closure after angioplasty.[34] Stent placement was successful in all 11 patients with non-Q-wave myocardial infarctions in two patients only; there was one additional instance of late-stent thrombosis at 3 months. DeFeyter reported 15 patients who received emergent Wallstents for acute occlusion following angioplasty, which was suspected to be on a basis other than thrombosis.[35] Implantation was technically successful in all patients, but nine patients underwent early emergency or semielective surgery, and two other patients had subacute thrombosis with infarction. Patients in both these series were treated with intracoronary urokinase in addition to heparin and aspirin after stent placement.

Most recently, Roubin described the results of emergency stenting in 115 patients receiving a balloon-expandable stainless-steel wire device.[33] The majority of patients (90%) had impending or threatened closure with evidence of dissections, reduced flow, and ischemia. Only 10% of patients had total vascular occlusion at the time of stenting. Initially successful stenting with a satisfactory arterial lumen was achieved in 93% ofattempts. Major complications included death (2%), myocardial infarction (16%), CABG (4%), and subacute thrombosis (8%).

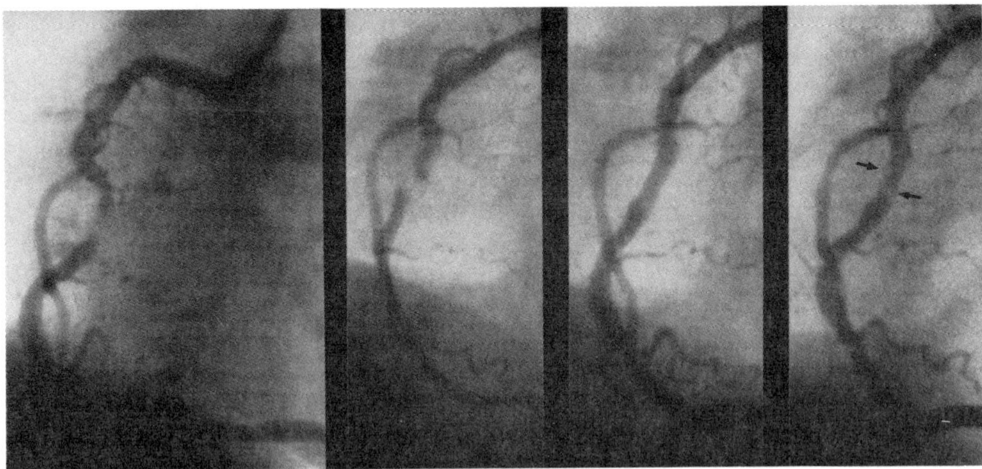

Figure 6: *Angiographic example of a patient with (from left to right): eccentric mid-right coronary artery lesion, development of intracoronary thrombus after conventional balloon angioplasty just prior to vessel occlusion, initial reestablishment of flow with intracoronary stenting, development of intraluminal filling defects (arrows) consistent with thrombus on the final poststent angiogram 30 minutes after stenting. This patient developed subacute stent thrombosis 2 days later despite therapeutic anticoagulation with heparin and suffered a myocardial infarction. (From,[25] with permission).*

Overall, the results of emergency stenting for failed angioplasty have been remarkably similar, with all three of the stent designs described above. High initial success rates with vessel salvage have been tempered by a subsequent need for emergency surgery or the development of other major complications, often in the setting of subacute thrombosis. Despite these problems, the majority of patients were able to avoid both initial complications and the need for late bypass surgery. In short-term follow-up, restenosis rates in patients receiving emergency stents have varied. In our series, the overall restenosis rate (> 50%–diameter stenosis) assessed in 85% of eligible patients was 23%, and was highest (43%) in vessels with true acute occlusion, but this difference was not statistically significant.[31] Roubin reported an overall restenosis rate of 41%.[33] Whether these rates are significantly lower than the high rates (81% and 55%) previously reported by Ba'albaki et al[40] and Cavallini et al[15] respectively, in patients with acute closure and successful reopening with conventional balloon angioplasty will require further study.

Comparison With Other Nonsurgical Modalities

A number of other nonsurgical modalities have been used to salvage failed angioplasty procedures. These include prolonged balloon inflations with standard or autoperfusion balloons, intracoronary thrombolytic agents, laser balloons, and atherectomy. In one preliminary study of the impact of several of these treatments on the management of acute occlusion, they appeared to lower the incidence of myocardial infarction and in-hospital CABG compared with an historical control group prior to the availability of the newer devices.[41]

In most cases of acute vessel closure after angioplasty, intracoronary thrombus is a major factor. In our own experience, thrombus complicated 6% of angioplasty procedures, and was occlusive in the majority of these cases.[13] Retrospectively, we examined treatment strategies including conservative management, redilation, and intracoronary urokinase in these patients, and demonstrated an overall major complication rate of 31%. Predictors of a good result without complications included the use of preprocedure antiplatelet therapy, an initial activated clotting time greater than 300 seconds, and rapid administration of urokinase when thrombus appeared.[13] The ideal dosing regimen for intracoronary urokinase in this setting is not clear and requires further investigation; one investigation with successful results used a mean of 150,000 units administered over 30 minutes.[25] Gulba and colleagues used a combination of intracoronary and intravenous recombinant tissue-type plasminogen activator to treat 27 patients with thrombotic occlusion after angioplasty.[26] Although successful reopening of the vessel was achieved in most patients, more than 50% developed early reocclusion, and could be identified by a failure of thrombin-antithrombin III complex levels to decrease.[26] The Stack autoperfusion catheter (Advanced Cardiovascular Systems, Mountain View, CA) allows prolonged balloon inflations (10 to 30 minutes) with minimal ischemia by passive perfusion of the distal coronary bed through multiple catheter side holes.[42] In 22 patients with either acute occlusion or obstructive dissection, Saenz and colleagues inflated a perfusion balloon for 11.3 min. (range 3 to 20 minutes) with improvement in angiographic appearance and flow.[27] Only one patient required surgery, but six patients(27%) had evidence of myocardial infarction. Similar results in patients with coronary dissection were also obtained by Leitschuh in a preliminary report.[28] Finally, the perfusion balloon has been used for prolonged (12 hours) inflations with good results in several cases.[43]

Laser-balloon angioplasty used a Nd:YAG laser to heat an inflated balloon and had the potential to weld arterial dissections, dessicate thrombi, and reduce the elastic properties of a stretched artery.[44] Although this technique is no longer available, in a preliminary report of a multicenter trial with this device in 21 patients, with acute occlusion due to dissection (12 patients), thrombus (eight patients), or both (one patient), laser-balloon angioplasty was able to reestablish flow, and emergency surgery was avoided in 20 of the 21 patients.[29]

Directional coronary atherectomy with the Simpson Atherocath (Devices for Vascular Interventions, Inc., Redwood City, CA) was recently approved by the FDA for clinical use. This device allows cutting and extraction of tissue and, theoretically, could be useful in the management of failed PTCA. Whitlow and colleagues described 22 patients with dissection (n = 12), thrombus (n =

1), or occlusion (n = 9) in whom atherectomy was used successfully in 82%. However, CABG was needed in 18%, and coronary perforation occurred in one patient with an extensive dissection.[30] This technique is also limited by the need to change guide catheters and femoral sheaths prior to insertion of the atherectomy device.

Examination of Table 2 which lists the results with several different interventions used to bailout unsuccessful PTCA procedures shows that initial restoration of vessel flow can be achieved in the majority of patients. Late success, however, is often lower due to subsequent complications. Unfortunately, more specific comparisons between the various interventions cannot be made in these highly selected series using different techniques and definitions.

Summary and Recommendations

Role of Stenting in Failed Percutaneous Transluminal Coronary Angioplasty

In elective situations, the Palmaz-Schatz balloon-expandable intracoronary stent has been demonstrated to have both high safety and efficacy. Stents have been implanted in more than 700 patients in United States centers participating in its investigation, with successful placement in 96% of attempts and a low rate of complications including death any time postimplant (1.5%), emergency surgery (3.4%), myocardial infarction (1.9%), and occlusion (including subacute thrombosis) (6.0%).[45]

In emergency situations, stent implantation is most likely to improve the results of a failed PTCA procedure when failure is due to intimal dissection or elastic recoil, rather than thrombosis. When PTCA failure is due to an obstructive dissection flap, stenting can seal the dissection, prevent occlusion of the vascular lumen, and protect against further propagation of the dissection. When PTCA failure is due to elastic recoil, a deployed stent may forcefully oppose the recoil. We have demonstrated successful stent deployment in 98% of 56 patients with PTCA failure, with successful initial procedure salvage in 90% of patients.[31]

On the other hand, stenting is less likely to be effective in managing a PTCA failure caused by thrombosis since the stent itself is a thrombogenic device and placement in a thrombotic site may exacerbate the problem. This may explain the high subacute thrombosis rate associated with emergent placement (16%) compared with elective use (6%). The likelihood of subsequent thrombosis may be partially predicted by the type of situation prompting emergent stenting, and by the development of angiographically-visible nonocclusive thrombus shortly after stent implantation. We found such thrombus in 44% of patients, and 13% of patients without subacute thrombosis (P = 0.03)[31] (Table 4). Future work should be directed toward developing better and more specific anticoagulation regimens, and toward design refinements which might reduce the tendency of stents for thrombosis.

The overall impact of stenting on early and late outcome of patients after failed PTCA and comparison with other modalities can only be inferred by examining reported outcomes in similar patient populations. In general, it appears that stenting can restore vessel patency in a very high proportion of failed PTCA procedures, but the late success rate falls due to subacute stent thrombosis. Comparisons between other modalities and other types of stents are limited by differences in vessel selection and size, the cause of PTCA failure, the use of thrombolytic agents and different anticoagulation regimens, and the use of other interventions prior to stenting.

Guidelines for Use

Following a failed PTCA procedure, several factors should be considered in the decision to use a stent for salvage (Table 5). Since stenting is more likely to be successful if the cause of failure is dissection or elastic recoil rather than thrombosis, an attempt should be made to determine the cause of failure. This determination is often difficult angiographically, and may be better assessed in the future with other imaging technologies.[18] However, if an initially good PTCA result is seen to develop progressive intraluminal filling defects, stent implantation should be avoided in favor of redilation and administration of intracoronary urokinase.[13]

Table 5.
Guidelines for Emergent Stenting after Failed PTCA

1. Determine cause, if possible, of failure
   a. Avoid stent use if primary vessel thrombosis
   b. Consider stent for dissection or elastic recoil
2. Maximize prestent anticoagulation
   a. Insure that aspirin was given pre-PTCA
   b. Administer heparin to ACT > 350 s.
   c. Administer LMW dextran (10%) with 500 ml bolus and continuous infusion (100 ml/h).
3. Anatomical considerations
   a. Location, size, length, tortuosity, side branches of target site
   b. Ease of delivery, choice of guide catheter
   c. Number of stents to completely seal dissection
   d. Minimize residual stenosis
4. Poststent considerations
   a. Prolonged angiographic observation (30–45 m)
      1. Aggressive treatment of intrastent thrombus
      2. Consider early surgery if suboptimal stent result
   b. Careful anticoagulation management
      1. Minimize heparin interruption for sheath removal
      2. Keep PTT high (~100 s)
      3. Overlap heparin with therapeutic PT for 48 h
   c. Prolonged in-hospital monitoring

PTCA = percutaneous transluminal coronary angioplasty; ACT = activated clotting time; LMW = low-molecular weight; PT= prothrombin time; PTT = partial thromboplastin time.

Once the decision to implant a stent is made, consideration should be given to the anticoagulation status of the patient. Heparin should be administered to maintain an activated clotting time greater than 300 seconds, and low-molecular weight dextran (10%) should be administered intravenously. We give a bolus infusion of 500 ml per hour over 30 to 60 minutes, followed by a continuous infusion of 100 ml per hour for 5 additional hours. The patient's medical record should be reviewed to confirm that preprocedural aspirin was given.

In placement of the stent, the operators should review the anatomy of the lesion in terms of potential stent location, ease of delivery, length of lesion, side branches, vessel tortuosity, and type of guide catheter backup needed (see Chapter 2). During stent placement, it is important to completely seal dissections both to prevent further propagation and because residual dissection poststenting has been associated with subacute thrombosis (Chapter 4). After stent placement, it should be fully expanded with an oversized balloon, if necessary, to minimize the residual stenosis in order to maximize flow and reduce the tendency for thrombosis.[31]

We recommend a prolonged period (30 to 45 minutes) of angiographic observation in the catheterization laboratory following successful emergency stenting. The development of even a small amount of intrastent thrombus during the observation period should be treated aggressively with intracoronary urokinase. Some investigators recommend a prolonged intracoronary urokinase infusion with an infusion wire or catheter in this situation. Patients with a suboptimal stent result due to residual dissection or thrombus are at greater than usual risk for subacute thrombosis, and consideration should be given to using the stent as a bridge to bypass surgery rather than as a permanent solution to the problem of failed PTCA. Follow-up angiography 24 hours after stent placement, before sheath removal, may sometimes be helpful in deciding whether to proceed with surgery.

Careful attention must be paid to the management of patients' anticoagulation status after emergent stenting. Heparin should be discontinued as briefly as possible for sheath removal. Our practice is to discontinue heparin for 2 to 3 hours, and remove the sheaths when the activated clotting time falls to 175 seconds. Heparin is reinstituted 30 minutes after hemostasis is achieved with a small bolus (2000 to 3000 units). The partial thromboplastin time should be compulsively monitored and maintained at a high level (100 seconds), if possible. Warfarin should be administered immediately and heparin should be continued for 48 hours after a therapeutic prothrombin time is achieved.[46] Finally, patients should be monitored in the hospital for 7 days poststenting to minimize the risk of subacute thrombosis occurring outside the hospital. The management of subacute thrombosis is discussed in Chapter 8.

REFERENCES

1. O'Keefe JH, Rutherford BD, McConahay DR, Johnson WL, Giorgi LV, Ligon RW, Shimshak TM, Hartzler GO: Multivessel coronary angioplasty from 1980–1989:

procedural results and long-term outcome. *J Am Coll Cardiol* 1990; 16:1097–1102.

2. Cowley MJ, Dorros G, Kelsey SF, van Raden M, Detre KM: Acute coronary events associated with percutaneous transluminal coronary angioplasty. *Am J Cardiol* 1984; 53:12C-16C.
3. Shiu MF, Silverton NP, Oakley D, Cumberland D: Acute coronary occlusion during percutaneous transluminal coronary angioplasty. *Br Heart J* 1985; 54:129–133.
4. Simpfendorfer C, Belardi J, Bellamy G, Galan K, Franco I, Hollman J: Frequency, management, and follow-up of patients with acute coronary occlusions after percutaneous transluminal coronary angioplasty. *Am J Cardiol* 1987; 59:267–269.
5. Ellis SG, Roubin GS, King SB, Douglas JS, Weintraub WS, Thomas RG, Cox WR: Angiographic and clinical predictors of acute closure after native vessel coronary angioplasty. *Circulation* 1988; 77:372–379.
6. Meyerovitz MF, Friedman PL, Ganz P, Selwyn AP, Levin DC: Acute occlusion developing during or immediately after percutaneous transluminal coronary angioplasty: nonsurgical treatment. *Cardiovasc Radiol* 1988; 169:491–494.
7. Sinclair IN, McCabe CH, Sipperly ME, Baim DS: Predictors, therapeutic options and long-term outcome of abrupt reclosure. *Am J Cardiol* 1988; 61:61G-66G.
8. Steffenino G, Meier B, Finci L, Velebit V, von Segesser L, Faidutti S, Rutishauser W: Acute complications of elective coronary angioplasty: a review of 500 consecutive procedures. *Br Heart J* 1988;59:151–158.
9. Detre KM, Holmes DR, Holubkov R, Cowley MJ, Bourassa MG, Faxon DP, Dorros GR, Bentivoglio LG, Kent KM, Myler RK: Incidence and consequences of periprocedural occlusion. *Circulation* 1990; 82:739–750.
10. deFeyter PJ, van den Brand M, Laarman G, van Domburg R, Serruys PW, Suryapranata H: Acute coronary artery occlusion during and after percutaneous transluminal coronary angioplasty. *Circulation* 1991; 83:927–936.
11. Lincoff AM, Popma JJ, Ellis SG, Hacker JA, Topol EJ: Abrupt vessel closure complicating coronary angioplasty: clinical, angiographic and therapeutic profile. *J Am Coll Cardiol* 1992; 19:926–935.
12. Gaul G, Hollman J, Simpfendorfer C, Franco I: Acute occlusion in multiple lesion coronary angioplasty: frequency and management. *J Am Coll Cardiol* 1989; 13: 283–288.
13. Vaitkus PT, Herrmann HC, Laskey WK: Management and immediate outcome of patients developing intracoronary thrombus during percutaneous transluminal coronary angioplasty. *Am Heart J* 1992; 124(1):1–8.
14. Breadlau CE, Roubin GS, Leimgruber PP, Douglas JS, King SB, Gruentzig AR: In-hospital morbidity and mortality in patients undergoing elective coronary angioplasty. *Circulation* 1985; 72:1044–1052.
15. Cavallini C, Giommi L, Franceschini E, Risicia G, Olivari Z, Marton F, Cuzzato V: Coronary angioplasty in single-vessel complex lesions: short- and long-term outcome and factors predicting acute coronary occlusions. *Am Heart J* 1991; 122:44–49.
16. Ischinger J, Gruentzig AR, Meier B, Galan K: Coronary dissection and total coronary occlusion associated with percutaneous transluminal coronary angioplasty: significance of initial angiographic morphology of coronary stenoses. *Circulation* 1986; 74:1371–1378.
17. Goldbaum T, DiSciascio G, Cowley MJ, Vetrovec GW: Early occlusion following successful coronary angioplasty: clinical and angiographic observations. *Cathet Cardiovasc Diagn* 1989; 17:22–27.
18. Shapiro TA, Herrmann HC: Coronary angiography and interventional cardiology. *Curr Opin Radiol* 1992; 4:55–64.
19. Isner JM, Rosenfield K, Losordo DW, Rose I, Langevin RE, Razvi S, Kosowsky BD: Combination balloon-ultrasound imaging catheter for percutaneous transluminal angioplasty: validation of imaging, analysis of recoil, and identification of plaque fracture. *Circulation* 1991; 84:739–754.

20. Talley JD, Weintraub WS, Roubin GS, Douglas JS, Anderson V, Jones EL, Morris DC, Liberman HA, Craver JM, Guyton RA, King SB: Failed elective percutaneous transluminal coronary angioplasty requiring coronary artery bypass surgery. *Circulation* 1990; 82:1203–1213.
21. Connor AR, Vlietstra RE, Schaff HV, Ilstrup DM, Orszulak TA: Early and late results of coronary artery bypass after failed angioplasty. *J Thorac Cardiovasc Surg* 1988; 96:191–197.
22. Page US, Okies JE, Colburn LQ, Bigelow JC, Salomon NW, Krause AH: Percutaneous transluminal coronary angioplasty. *J Thorac Cardiovasc Surg* 1986; 92: 847–852.
23. Reul GJ, Cooley DA, Hallman GL, Duncan JM, Livesay JJ, Frazier OH, Ott DA, Angelina P, Massumi A, Mathur VS: Coronary artery bypass for unsuccessful percutaneous transluminal coronary angioplasty. *J Thorac Cardiovasc Surg* 1984; 88: 685–694.
24. Schomig A,Dietz R, Kubbler W, Hsu E, Kranzhofer R: Outcome after emergency implantation of coronary stents. *J Am Coll Cardiol* 1992; 19:198A. Abstract.
25. Schieman G, Cohen BM, Kozina J, Erickson JS, Podolin RA, Peterson KL, Ross J, Buchbinder M: Intracoronary urokinase for intracoronary thrombus accumulation complicating percutaneous transluminal coronary angioplasty in acute ischemic syndromes. *Circulation* 1990; 82:2052–2060.
26. Gulba DC, Daniel WG, Simon R, Jost S, Barthels M, Amende I, Rafflenbeul W, Lichtlen PR: Role of thrombolysis and thrombin in patients with acute coronary occlusion during percutaneous transluminal coronary angioplasty. *Am Coll Cardiol* 1990; 16:563–568.
27. Saenz CB, Schwartz KM, Slysh SJ, Palanca K, Curry, RC: Experience with the use of coronary autoperfusion catheter during complicated angioplasty. *Cathet Cardiovasc Diagn* 1990; 20:276–278.
28. Leitschuh ML, LaRosa D, Currier JW, Mills RM, Jacobs AK, Ruocco NA, Faxon DP: The "Stack perfusion catheter" improves outcome following dissection during coronary angioplasty. *J Am Coll Cardiol* 1990; 15:250A. Abstract.
29. Ferguson JJ, Dear WE, Leatherman LL, Safian RD, King SB, Douglas JS, Spears JR: A multicenter trial of laser balloon angioplasty for abrupt closure following PTCA. *J Am Coll Cardiol* 1990; 15:25A. Abstract.
30. Whitlow PL, Robertson GC, Rowe MH, Douglas JS, Cowley MJ, Kereiakes DJ, Smucker ML, Hartzler GO, Hinohara T: Directional coronary atherectomy for failed percutaneous transluminal coronary angioplasty. *Circulation* 1990; 82:III-1.
31. Herrmann HC, Buchbinder M, Clemen MW, Fischman D, Goldberg S, Leon MB, Schatz RA, Tierstein P, Walker CM, Hirshfeld JW: Emergent use of balloon-expandable coronary artery stenting for failed PTCA. *Circulation* 1992; 86:812–819.
32. Haude M, Erbel R, Straub U, Dietz U, Schatz R, Meyer J: Results of intracoronary stents for management of coronary dissection after balloon angioplasty. *Am J Coll Cardiol* 1991; 67:691–696.
33. Roubin GS, Cannon AD, Agrawal SK, Macander PJ, Dean LS, Baxley WA, Breland J: Intracoronary stenting for acute and threatened closure complicating percutaneous transluminal coronary angioplasty. *Circulation* 1992; 85:916–927.
34. Sigwart U, Urban P, Golf S, Kaufmann U, Imbert C, Fischer A, Kappenberger L: Emergency stenting for acute occlusion after coronary balloon angioplasty. *Circulation* 1988; 78:1121–1127.
35. deFeyter PJ, DeScheerder I, van den Brand M, Laarman G, Suryapranata H, Serruys PW: Emergency stenting for refractory acute coronary artery occlusion during coronary angioplasty. *Am J Cardiol* 1990; 66:1147–1150.
36. Kimura T, Nosaka H, Yokoi H, Hamasaki N, Nobuyoshi M: Emergency coronary stenting for abrupt closure and dissection after balloon angioplasty. *J Am Coll Cardiol* 1992; 19:198A. Abstract.
37. Fajadet J, Jenny D, Guabliumi G, Cassagneau B, Robert G, Jordan C, Flores M,

Marco J: Immediate and late outcome of bailout coronary stenting. *J Am Coll Cardiol* 1992; 19:109A. Abstract.

38. Penn IM, Brown RIG, MacDonald R, Ricci D, Almond D, Burton J, O'Neill B, Galligan L, Foley JB, Murray-Parsons N, White J, Slivocka J: Stent complications are dependent on the "stent environment: Multicentre Canadian Experience. *J Am Coll Cardiol* 1992; 19:47A. Abstract.
39. Kiemeneij F, Laarman G, Suwarganda J, van der Wieken R: Emergent coronary stenting after failed coronary angioplasty: immediate and mean term results with the Palmaz-Schatz stent. *J Am Coll Cardiol* 1992; 19:47A. Abstract.
40. Ba'albaki HA, Weintraub WS, Tao X, Ghazzal ZMB, Liberman HA, Douglas JS, King SB: Restenosis after acute closure and successful reopening: implications for new devices. *Circulation* 1990; 82:III-314. Abstract.
41. Scott NA, Weintraub WS, Carlin SF, Tao X, Hearn JA, Lembo NJ, Douglas JS, King SB: Acute closure during PTCA: improved management with intracoronary stents, laser balloons and prolonged inflation. *J Am Coll Cardiol* 1992; 19:93A. Abstract.
42. Hinohara T, Simpson JB, Phillips HR, Stack RS: Transluminal intracoronary reperfusion catheter: a device to maintain coronary perfusion between failed coronary angioplasty and emergency coronary bypass surgery. *J Am Coll Cardiol* 1988; 11: 977–982.
43. Little T: Prolonged coronary splinting in the management of acute coronary closure. *Cathet Cardiovasc Diagn* 1992; 25:213–217.
44. Jenkins RD, Spears JR: Laser balloon angioplasty: a new approach to abrupt coronary occlusion and chronic restenosis. *Circulation* 1990; 81(suppl IV):IV-101-IV-108.
45. Leon MB, Kent KM, Baim DS, Walker CM, Clemen MW, Buchbinder M, Heuser RR, Curry C, Schatz R: Comparison of stent implantation in native coronaries and saphenous vein grafts. *J Am Coll Cardiol* 1992; 19:263A. Abstract.
46. Hirsch J: Oral anticoagulant drugs. *N Engl J Med* 1991; 324:1865–1875.

CHAPTER 7

Balloon-Expandable Stent Implantation in Saphenous Vein Grafts

Martin B. Leon
Shing-Chiu Wong
Augusto D. Pichard

Conventional balloon angioplasty in patients with saphenous vein graft disease often yields unpredictable acute angiographic results, a higher frequency of intraprocedural complications (including distal embolization), and increased propensity for restenosis.[1-5] Therefore, alternative transcatheter techniques for the purpose of achieving safe and predictable acute angiographic results and lower restenosis frequency have been under intensive investigation.

Over the past 5 years, balloon-expandable stents have found clinical application in a variety of patient subsets with native coronary disease: 1) abrupt or threatened abrupt closure; 2) suboptimal PTCA results with significant residual stenosis; 3) unfavorable or unusual lesion morphology at high risk for PTCA complications; 4) to reduce the frequency of restenosis in de novo lesions or recurrent restenotic lesions.[6-11] More recently, preliminary observations have indicated that stents may be a useful therapy in treating patients with aortocoronary saphenous vein graft disease. The use of a self-expanding metallic stent in patients with stenoses within the shaft portion of saphenous vein grafts indicated high procedural success, few complications, and a lower than expected frequency of restenosis.[12,13]

This chapter outlines the multicenter experience using the Johnson & Johnson Interventional System (JJIS) balloon-expandable Palmaz-Schatz stent (Johnson & Johnson Intervenional Systems, Inc., Warren, NJ) in patients with saphenous vein graft disease who fulfill specific study inclusion criteria.

From: Herrmann HC, Hirshfeld JW, eds. *Clinical Use of the Palmaz-Schatz Intracoronary Stent.* Futura Publishing Company, Inc., Mount Kisco, NY, © 1993.

Study Design

Seventeen institutions participated in this multicenter trial with the purpose of examining the safety and efficacy of balloon-expandable stent implantation in the shaft portion of aortocoronary saphenous vein grafts (3 to 5 mm in diameter), at focal lesion sites (less than 15 mm-axial length), with good distal runoff into the native vasculature. The investigators were encouraged to avoid true aorto-ostial lesions, distal anastomotic site lesions, diffuse disease (greater than 15 mm in length), and either smaller, (less than 3 mm) or larger (greater than 5 mm) vein-graft diameter, which would be poorly suited to the current coronary-stent design.

In all patients, the JJIS Palmaz-Schatz coronary stent was employed. The technique of stenting for saphenous vein grafts is similar to previous experience in native coronaries. The lesion is crossed using a .014-inch guidewire, and predilatation is performed, usually using undersized balloon catheters. Next, the stent-delivery system is placed across the lesion site, the sheath is retracted into the guiding catheter, and the stent is deployed with a single-balloon inflation to nominal pressures. As needed, postdilatation is performed, often with larger balloon catheters to achieve the best "match" of stent size to contiguous reference vessel segments.

The pharmacologic regimen used before, during, and after stent implantation is identical to the regimen used in native coronary arteries (see Chapter 2). Importantly, patients are carefully selected and the candidates have no contraindications to either the antiplatelet therapy or prolonged systemic anticoagulation.

Results of Stenting in Saphenous Vein Grafts

Patient Demographics

In 626 consecutive patients, stent implantation was attempted using the JJIS balloon-expandable stent-delivery system. Patient characteristics are described in Table 1. Most patients (85%) were male with a mean age of 66 ± 9 years. The mean age of the vein grafts receiving stents was 8.9 ± 4.2 years (Table 1).

Stent Delivery and Lesion Characteristics

Of the 626 patient cohort, the overall deployment success rate was 98.7%. Eight patients had unsuccessful stent deployment. In addition, within the group of 618 patients who had successful stent delivery, 13 patients had at least one failed attempt before subsequent successful stent deployment. In the

Table 1.
Patient Demographics (n = 626 patients)

Age (range)	66 ± 9 years (39–88 years)
Male	85%
Hypertension	59%
Diabetes	28%
Cholesterol > 200	71%
Hx Smoking	72%
Family Hx CAD	65%
Angina Status:	
CCVS 0	3%
CCVS 1	2%
CCVS 2	8%
CCVS 3	22%
CCVS 4	65%
Prior PTCA:	
1	38%
2	20%
> 2	6%
SVG age	8.9 ± 4.2 years (0.08–21.7 years)
LV ejection fraction	49 ± 14%

eight patients with unsuccessful stent deployment, six stents were retrieved. In one patient, two stents were deployed proximally and one embolized into the periphery. In another patient, poststent dilatation with a large (5.0 mm) balloon catheter resulted in graft rupture with associated cardiac tamponade.

In patients with successful stent delivery, single stents were implanted in 505 patients (82%), multiple single stents were implanted in 75 patients (12%), overlapping tandem stents in 35 patients (6%), and in one patient, three single and two overlapping tandem stents were implanted.

Lesion characteristics for the 618 patients with successful stent implantation are summarized in Table 2. Of interest, 28 of the 41 patients with thrombus identified prior to stent implantation were treated with intragraft thrombolytic agents. Neither the presence of thrombus at the lesion site nor the use of

Table 2.
Lesion Characteristics (618 patients)

Reference Vessel Diameter	3.6 ± 0.7 mm
Maximum % Diameter Stenosis	82 ± 12%
Minimum Lumen Diameter	0.7 ± 0.5 mm
Lesion Length	7.6 ± 4.9 mm
Thrombus at Lesion (% of patients)	6.6%

intragraft thrombolytic agents influenced deployment success or acute angiographic results after stent implantation.

Acute Angiographic Results

In general, balloon-expandable stent implantation resulted in marked improvement in lumen dimensions with sharp lumen contours, brisk flow, and minimal residual stenosis. This was true, even in situations where complex lesion morphologies were treated and prestent angioplasty results were suboptimal (Fig. 1). Percent-diameter stenosis at the lesion site decreased from 82% pretreatment, to 45% after predilatation PTCA, and to 7% poststent implantation (Fig. 2). Similarly, minimum lumen diameter increased from 0.7 mm pretreatment to 3.4 mm poststent placement (Fig. 2).

In 43 patients (7%), angiographic dissection was present after predilatation PTCA and before stent implantation. Dissections were eliminated in 35 of these patients (81%), but new dissections were noted poststent in an additional eight patients (1.3%) (Fig. 3).

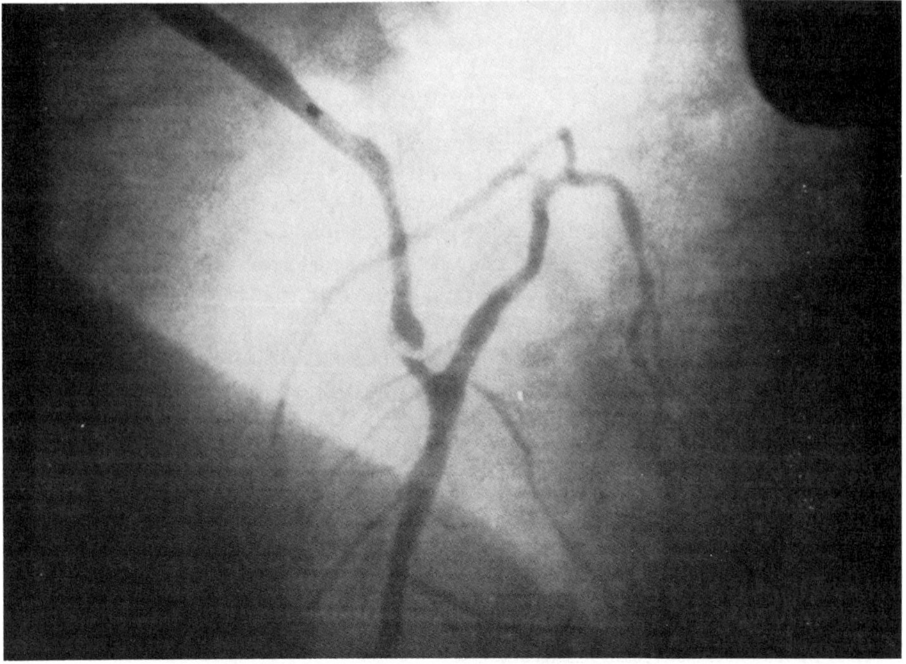

Figure 1: *Coronary cineangiograms showing pretreatment stenosis* **(A)**, postballoon angioplasty **(B)**, and poststent implantation **(C)**, in the distal shaft portion of a saphenous vein graft to the left anterior descending artery. Note the marked improvement in lumen dimensions after stenting, despite the complex lesion morphology and poor response to conventional balloon angioplasty.

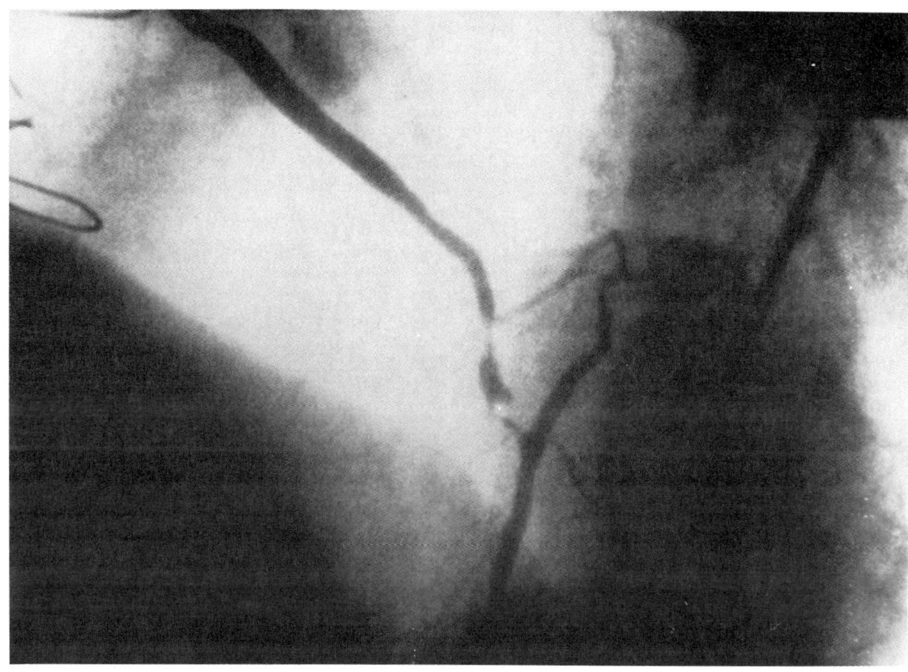

Figure 1B: *Postballoon angioplasty.*

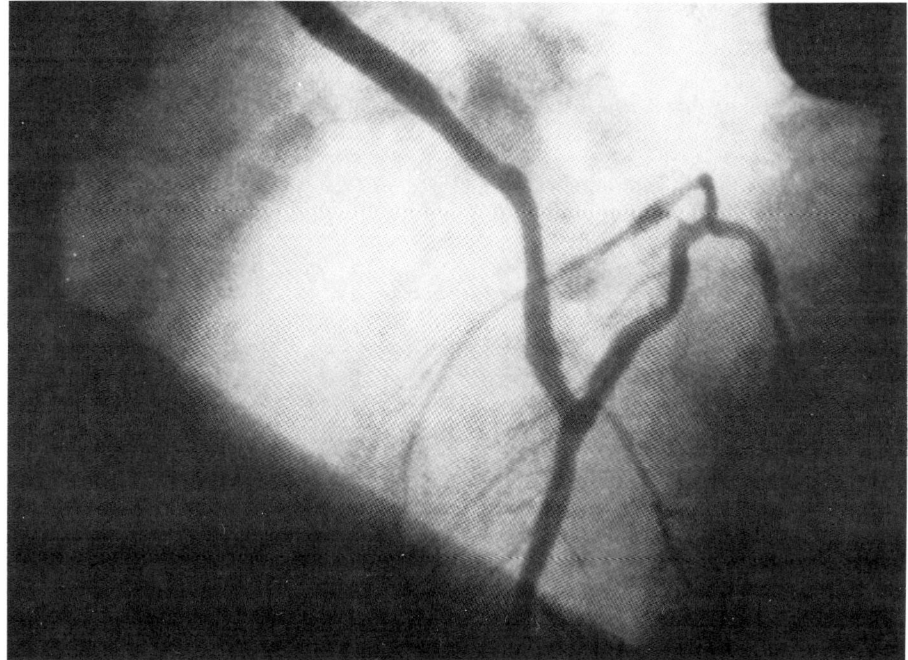

Figure 1C: *Poststent implantation.*

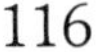

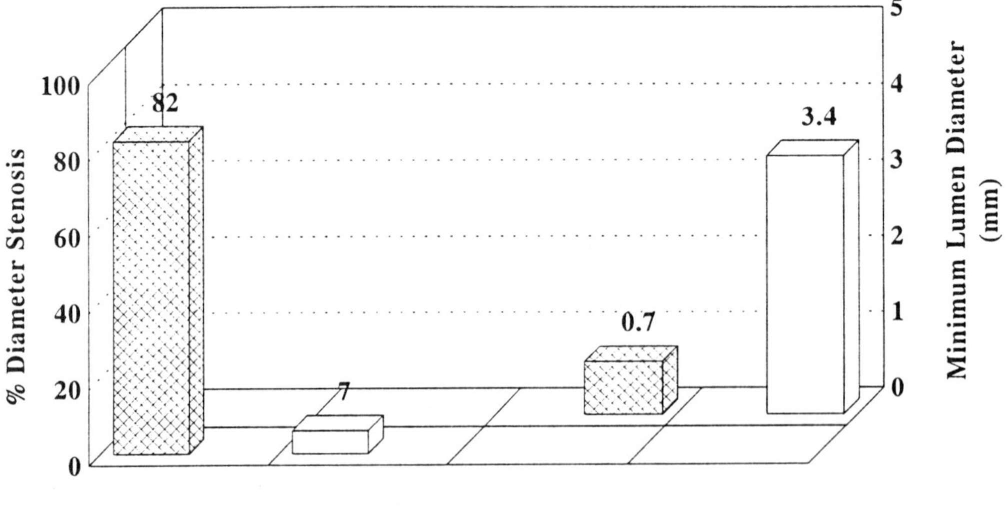

Figure 2: *Percent-diameter stenosis (left) and minimum lumen diameter (right) pre-treatment (hatched bars) and poststent implantation (open bars) for the entire patient cohort.*

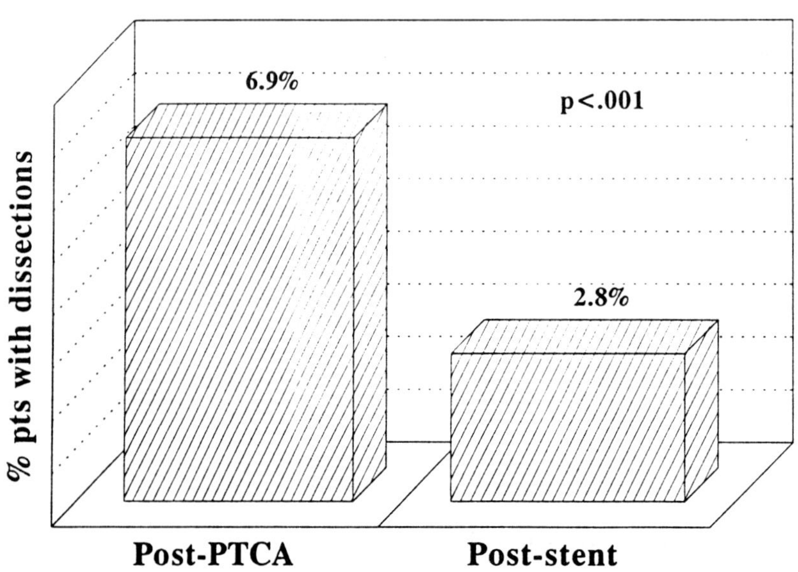

Figure 3: *Percent of patient with angiographic dissections after predilatation (before stent placement) and after subsequent stent implantation.*

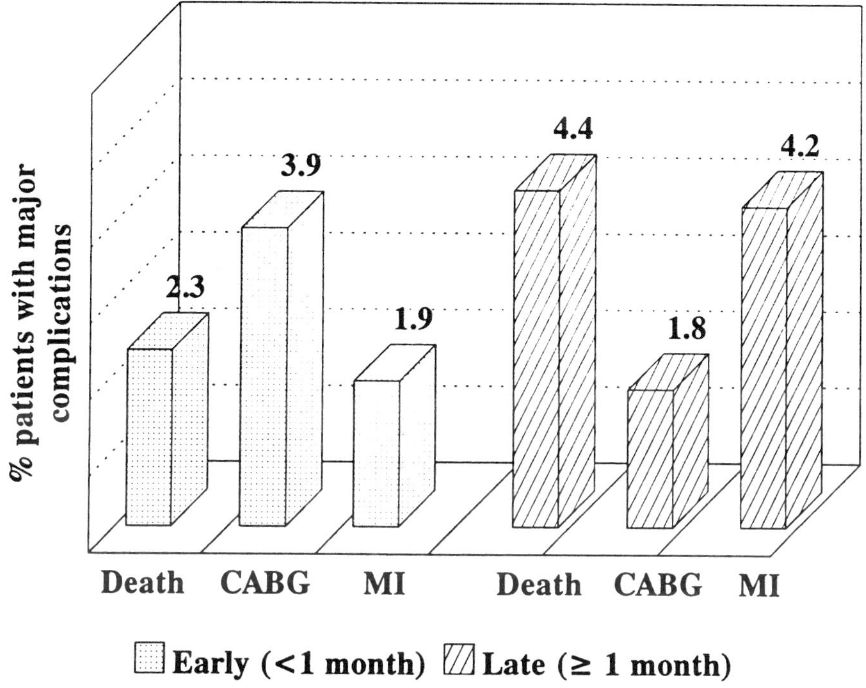

Figure 4: *The percent of patients with major complications occurring early (within 1 months of stent implantation) and late (after 1 month). Major complications include death, coronary artery bypass graft surgery, and myocardial infarction.*

Complications

The frequency of major complications (death, myocardial infarction, urgent coronary bypass graft surgery) occurring early (less than 1 month) and late (greater than 1 month) after stent implantation are shown in Figure 4. It bears noting that most of the early and late mortality was associated with intercurrent medical illnesses and were not stent-related deaths.

Acute or subacute thrombosis after stent implantation was described in eight patients (1.3%). The mean time to stent thrombosis from implantation was 5 days. Six events occurred in-hospital and two occurred out of hospital. None of the patients sustaining stent thrombosis events died, but three were referred for coronary bypass graft surgery, and four others sustained acute myocardial infarctions.

Embolization occurring during the procedure was noted in nine patients (1.5%). In five of these patients, creatine kinase elevations were present, indicating evidence of nontransmural infarction.

Bleeding complications associated with the intense anticoagulation regimen were numerous. Bleeding requiring transfusion (either at the access site or at other locations) occurred in 7.7% of patients. Surgical repair of the access

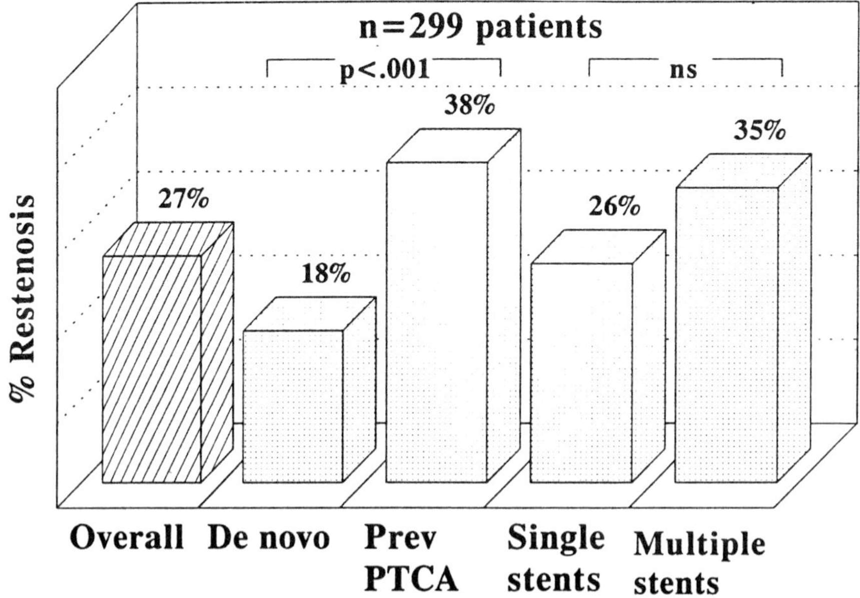

Figure 5: *Percent restenosis (> 50%–diameter narrowing during follow-up angiography) for 299 patients with follow-up angiographic examinations. Overall restenosis, and restenosis involving multiple subgroups are shown.*

site (due to arteriovenous fistula, pseudoaneurysm, or expanding hematoma) was required in 8% of patients. Cerebral hemorrhage temporally associated with intense anticoagulation during the early phases of stent implantation occurred in two patients (0.3%).

Restenosis

Angiographic follow-up was obtained in 299 patients, representing approximately half of those patients eligible for late angiography. The mean time to angiographic follow-up was 6.6 months. The overall restenosis frequency (≥ 50% diameter stenosis at follow-up angiography) was 27.4% (Fig. 5). Restenosis frequency was significantly lower in patients with de novo lesions (18%), compared with those with previous PTCA at the stent site (38%, $P < .001$) (Fig. 5). There were small statistically insignificant differences when comparing restenosis frequencies in single-stent versus multiple-stent implants (Fig. 5).

Discussion

This chapter attempts to summarize a consecutive patient experience detailing the results of stent implantation in patients with saphenous vein graft pathology. The data set represents a fairly homogeneous group of patients with focal lesions in the shaft segment of saphenous vein grafts which are 3 to 5 mm in diameter. These results cannot be extrapolated to diffuse disease within the vein graft shaft, aorto-ostial lesions, or distal anastomotic site lesions. Patients were severely symptomatic (87 % CCVS class III or IV), and 38% had prior PTCA at the treatment site. Deployment success was excellent (98.7% per patient), and acute stent-related complications were rare. The immediate angiographic findings indicate a dramatic improvement in minimum lumen diameter (from .7 mm to 3.4 mm), and a marked reduction in maximum percent-diameter stenosis (from 82% to 7%) after stent implantation. Similarly, PTCA-induced dissections prior to stent implantation were usually obliterated after stent placement.

Although this does not represent a randomized trial, follow-up angiography in almost 300 patients indicates an overall restenosis frequency less than 30%. There was a statistically significant difference in the restenosis frequency between de novo lesions (18%) and lesions which had been treated previously using PTCA (38%). Early and late major complications were acceptable, especially noting that many late morbid events were associated with intercurrent medical illnesses. Importantly, acute or subacute thrombosis in saphenous vein grafts receiving stents was surprisingly low compared to previous series of stents in native coronary arteries.[14,15] The reason for this difference is unclear, but may relate to the larger vein graft size, straight-shaft segment with better flow properties and no branch vessels, or intrinsic differences in thrombogenicity associated with the vascular biology of arterialized venous conduits. Nevertheless, this low frequency of stent-related thrombosis removes one of the obstacles to more widespread use of this technique in patients with saphenous vein graft lesions. Of note, although thrombosis frequency is low, bleeding complications associated with intensive systemic anticoagulation were disturbingly high. More than 15% of patients required transfusion for bleeding or surgical repair of the arteriotomy access site.

These data should be compared to previous historical series examining the efficacy of balloon angioplasty in patients with saphenous vein graft disease.[15,16] Undoubtedly, stent implantation results in a greater improvement in immediate angiographic results with predictable outcome compared to conventional PTCA. In only one patient of the reported stent series was the percent-diameter stenosis greater than 50% (53%) after stent implantation. Similarly, a final average percent-diameter stenosis of 7% for stent patients is substantially lower than any reported series of vein-graft shaft stenosis treated using PTCA techniques.[15,16] Another apparent difference between stent therapy and PTCA in saphenous vein graft lesions is the lower peripheral embolization frequency (1.5%) seen in stent patients. Perhaps, this is due to the "less aggressive" predilatation strategy with brief inflations using undersized balloons, followed by a single-balloon expansion for stent deployment. By minimizing balloon-vessel wall contact, the opportunity for lesion fragmentation and subsequent embolization may be reduced. In addition, the obvious scaffolding effect of the stent itself may, importantly, prevent plaque rupture and disintegration.

In the absence of a randomized trial, it is not possible to conclude that stent implantation reduces restenosis frequency. However, compared with historical PTCA series, the overall restenosis rate of 27% and the restenosis frequency in de novo lesions of 18% is most encouraging. Furthermore, the angiographic follow-up in the stent series was only 50%, and since the majority of nonstudied follow-up patients were asymptomatic, the "true" restenosis frequency may, in fact, be less than described in this report. Randomized trials in both de novo and restenosis patients with focal saphenous vein graft lesions are being planned now to answer this important question: Does stent implantation reduce restenosis frequency?

Conclusions

This report demonstrates that stent implantation in the shaft portion of aortocoronary saphenous vein grafts results in high delivery success, excellent acute procedure results, acceptable complications, and a lower than expected restenosis frequency. Stent thrombosis was a rare event and did not contribute to mortality. However, bleeding complications, especially at the arteriotomy access site, remain problematic and should be addressed in the future. The use of thromboresistant coatings on stents to minimize the need for aggressive systemic anticoagulation combined with local arteriotomy closure devices may significantly influence these bleeding events in years to come. These data provide hope that stent implantation may become the preferred treatment in patients with saphenous vein graft stenoses due to improved and predictable acute results combined with greater long-term patency.

REFERENCES

1. Douglas JS Jr, Greuntzig AR, King SB III, Hollman J, Ischinger T, Meier B, Craver JM, Jones EL, Waller JL, Bone DK, Guyton R: Percutaneous transluminal coronary angioplasty in patients with prior coronary bypass surgery. *J Am Coll Cardiol* 1983; 2:745–754.
2. Block PC, Cowley MJ, Kaltenbach M, Kent KM, Simpson J: Percutaneous angioplasty of stenosis of bypass grafts or of bypass graft anastomotic sites. *Am J Cardiol* 1984; 53:666–668.
3. Douglas J, Robinson K, Schlumpf M, Gruentzig Cardiovascular Center: Percutaneous transluminal angioplasty in aortocoronary venous graft stenoses: immediate results and complications. *J Am Coll Cardiol* 1986, 59:II-363.
4. Pinkerton CA, Slack JD, Orr CM, Vantassel JW, Smith ML: Percutaneous transluminal angioplasty in patients with prior myocardial revascularization surgery. *Am J Cardiol* 1988; 61:15G-22G.
5. Platko WP, Hollman J, Whitlow PL, Franco I: Percutaneous transluminal angioplasty of saphenous vein graft stenosis: long-term follow-up. *J Am Coll Cardiol* 1989; 14:1645–1650.

6. Fischman DL, Savage MP, Leon MB, Schatz RA, Ellis SG, Cleman MW, Teirstein P, Walker CM, Bailey S, Hirshfeld JW Jr, Goldberg S: Effect of intracoronary stenting on intimal dissection after balloon angioplasty: results of quantitative and qualitative coronary analysis. *J Am Coll Cardiol* 1991; 18:1445–1451.
7. Lincoff AM, Popma JJ, Ellis SG, Hacker JA, Topol EJ: Abrupt vessel closure complicating coronary angioplasty: clinical, angiographic and therapeutic profile. *J Am Coll Cardiol* 1992; 19:926–935.
8. Roubin GS, Cannon AD, Agrawal SK, Macander PJ, Dean LS, Baxley WA, Breland J: Intracoronary stenting for acute and threatened closure complicating percutaneous transluminal coronary angioplasty. *Circulation* 1992; 85:916–927.
9. Goy JJ, Sigwart U, Vogt P, Stauffer JC, Kappenberger L: Long-term clinical and angiographic follow-up of patients treated with the self-expanding coronary stent for acute occlusion during balloon angioplasty of the right coronary artery. *J Am Coll Cardiol* 1992; 19:1593–1596.
10. Carrozza JP Jr, Kuntz RE, Levine MJ, Pomerantz RM, Fishman RF, Mansour M, Gibson CM, Senerchia CC, Diver DJ, Safian RD, Baim DS: Angiographic and clinical outcome of intracoronary stenting: immediate and long-term results from a large single-center experience. *J Am Coll Cardiol* 1992; 20:328–337.
11. Teirstein PS, Schatz RA, Leon MB, Goldberg S, Ellis S, Baim D, Stratienko A, Shaknovich A: Should patients with discrete, de novo coronary stenoses undergo stenting as a primary procedure? Risk vs benefit. (abstract) *J Am Coll Cardiol* 1991; 2:280A. Abstract.
12. Urban P, Sigwart U, Golf S, Kaufmann U, Sadeghi H, Kappenberger L: Intravascular stenting for stenosis of aortocoronary venous bypass grafts. *J Am Coll Cardiol* 1989; 13:1085–1091.
13. Strauss BH, Serruys PW, Bertrand ME, Puel J, Meier B, Goy JJ, Kappenberger L, Rickards AF, Sigwart U: Quantitative angiographic follow-up of the coronary Wallstent in native vessels and bypass grafts (European Experience: March 1986 to March 1990). *Am J Cardiol* 1992; 69:475–481.
14. Schatz RA, Baim DS, Leon M, Ellis SG, Goldberg S, Hirshfeld JW, Cleman MW, Cabin HS, Walker C, Stagg J, Buchbinder M, Teirstein PS, Topol EJ, Savage M, Perez JA, Curry RC, Whitworth H, Sousa E, Tio FO, Almagor Y, Ponder R, Penn IM, Leonard B, Levine SL, Fish RD, Palmaz JC: Clinical experience with the Palmaz-Schatz coronary stent; initial results of a multicenter study. *Circulation* 1991; 83:148–161.
15. Leon MB, Kent KM, Baim DS, Walker CM, Cleman MW, Buchbinder M, Heuser RR, Curry C, Schatz RA, and JJIS Stent Investigators: Comparison of stent implantation in native coronaries and saphenous vein grafts. *J Am Coll Cardiol* 1992; 3; 263A.
16. Kussmaul WG III: Percutaneous angioplasty of coronary bypass grafts: an emerging consensus. *Cathet Cardiovasc Diagn* 1988; 15:1–4. Editorial.

IV

Management of Stent-Related Complications

CHAPTER 8

Coronary Stent Thrombosis

David L. Fischman
Michael P. Savage
Sheldon Goldberg

Coronary artery stenting has undergone extensive evaluation as a means to circumvent the two major limitations of coronary angioplasty: acute occlusion and late restenosis. Preliminary studies have demonstrated that stenting may be useful in these areas; however, this new technique remains limited by the occurrence of acute and subacute stent thrombosis.

Recent reports with different stent designs have shown various rates of stent thrombosis.[1–3] In one study of 105 patients treated with the self-expanding Wallstent, there was a 24% rate of thrombosis, with 21 of 25 occlusions occurring within 2 weeks after stent placement.[1] For the most part, these early thrombotic occlusions occurred despite vigorous anticoagulation. In addition, stent thrombosis frequently has serious consequences; the overall mortality in this series was 7.6%. If stents are to achieve their promise of optimizing the primary angioplasty result and reducing the restenosis risk, the issue of thrombogenicity must be addressed, and the risk of stent thrombosis reduced.

The purpose of this chapter is to review the results and risk of thrombosis in experimental and clinical trials with the balloon-expandable Palmaz-Schatz stent. In particular, we will examine the clinical and angiographic factors associated with increased thrombosis rates. The clinical insights which result from these experiences may help reduce the risk of acute occlusion after stent placement.

In Vivo Experimental Studies With the Palmaz-Schatz Stent

Early canine studies with the Palmaz-Schatz stent have demonstrated that following stent implantation, as with angioplasty, a complex process of healing

From: Herrmann HC, Hirshfeld JW, eds. *Clinical Use of the Palmaz-Schatz Intracoronary Stent.* Futura Publishing Company, Inc., Mount Kisco, NY, © 1993.

and reendothelialization occurs (see Chapter 1). As with any metallic implant, thrombogenicity was a major concern. Therefore, Palmaz et al tested the thrombogenicity of their balloon-expandable intraluminal stent in the canine model. Sixty-four dogs received stents in the hind leg (expanded with the size-range of human coronary arteries), treated with various anticoagulation levels, and evaluated by indium-labeled platelet scans and gross inspection (see Fig. 1).

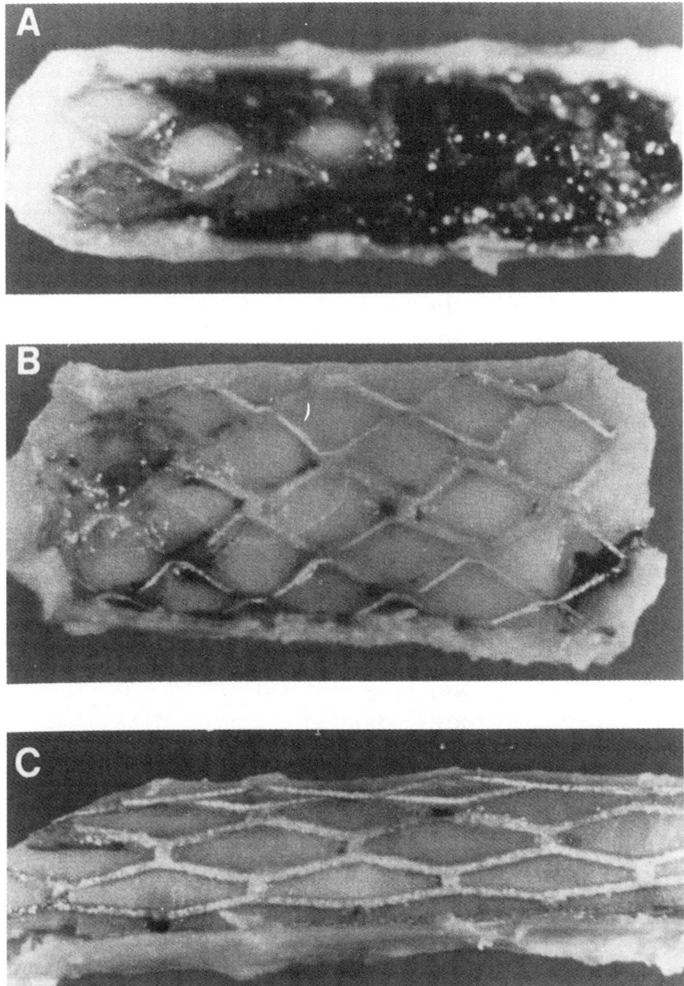

Figure 1: *The effect of various anticoagulation regimens on visible thrombus in the canine model. Panel* **A** is from an animal receiving no anticoagulation. Panel **B** represents treatment with heparin, aspirin, and dipyridamole. Panel **C** is treatment with dextran in addition to heparin, aspirin, and dipyridamole. Note the absence of thrombus with the addition of dextran. (Reproduced with permission from Schatz RA: A view of vascular stents. *Circulation* 1989; 79:445).

Stented animals treated with aspirin, dipyridamole, heparin, and low-molecular weight dextran developed less thrombus than stented controls and animals given various combinations of heparin, aspirin, and dipyridamole.[4] Based on these preliminary studies, it was concluded that dextran reduced the thrombogenicity and optimized neointimal growth by preventing uncontrolled platelet and thrombus deposition in these stainless-steel stents. In the first intracoronary use of stents, 20 stents were placed in the coronary arteries of dogs treated with aspirin, dipyridamole, low-molecular weight dextran, and heparin. All stents remained patent at a mean-time period of 18 months, with no incidence of acute thrombotic occlusion, myocardial infarction, or death in these animals.[5]

Clinical Trials

In November 1987, a multicenter clinical trial was initiated. The early phase of this study used a nonarticulated stent design which was subsequently modified by means of a central-bridging strut. Based on the results of thrombogenicity testing in animals, the following anticoagulation regimen was used in patients who underwent stent placement: aspirin (325 mg daily) and dipyridamole (75 mg T.I.D.) were begun at least 24 to 48 hours before stenting. All patients were treated with low-molecular weight dextran 40 (100 cc per hour intravenous) beginning 2 hours before stent deployment, and continued for a total dose of 1 liter. Heparin was given as an initial bolus in the catheterization laboratory, followed by intermittent boluses to maintain the activated clotting time 2 to 2.5 times control. After the procedure, heparin was continued to maintain the partial prothrombin time 1.5 to 2.5 times control for at least 24 hours. Dipyridamole was continued for 3 months, and aspirin was continued indefinitely. Coumadin was not included in the anticoagulation regimen of the first 39 patients. However, a high-stent thrombosis rate of 18% was observed in these patients and, therefore, coumadin was subsequently added to the anticoagulation regimen.[6] Currently, coumadin is initiated on the evening after the procedure, and adjusted to maintain a prothrombin time of 16 to 18 seconds for 1 month after which coumadin is discontinued.

Results and Predictors of Stent Thrombosis

Influence of Coumadin

Despite the use of coumadin, stent thrombosis has remained a major limitation of this device. From November 1988 through August 31, 1991, 983 patients underwent stenting of native coronary arteries with the Palmaz-Schatz stent in the United States. Of these 983 patients, 67 patients were not treated with coumadin, and stent thrombosis occurred in eight (11.9%). In the remaining 916 patients treated with coumadin, stent thrombosis occurred in 41 patients (4.5%). Overall, stent thrombosis occurred in 49 of 983 patients for an incidence of 5%. The mean-time course to this event was 6 days, with a range of 1 to 23 days. In all but one patient, stent thrombosis occurred beyond 24 hours after implantation.

Angiographic Predictors of Stent Thrombosis

To determine if factors other than coumadin were associated with thrombotic events, an angiographic evaluation of documented thrombotic events was performed at the core angiographic laboratory.[7] Qualitative and quantitative analyses were performed in 303 patients; 36 patients with documented stent thrombosis, and a control population of 267 patients without stent thrombosis. Angiography was performed at baseline, following conventional balloon angioplasty, and following stent placement in these patients. Quantitative analysis of digitized cineangiograms was performed using an automatic edge-detection program with paired orthogonal views. Qualitative analysis was performed by a panel of experienced angiographers. For purposes of this study, thrombus was defined as an intraluminal-filling defect surrounded by contrast (for subtotal occlusion), or a total occlusion, either with a convex border or delayed contrast staining.

Table 1 shows the clinical characteristics of the patients with and without stent thrombosis. No difference was noted in the patient populations with respect to sex, age, incidence of previous angioplasty, or angina class. Of note, approximately 40% had unstable angina at rest in both groups.

Baseline lesion characteristics and their association with stent thrombosis are depicted in Table 2. Specifically, no difference was noted in patients with and without stent thrombosis with respect to lesion eccentricity, calcification,

Table 1.
Patient Characteristics

	Thrombosis	*No Thrombosis*	*p*
No. of Patients	36	267	
male (%)	72	79	ns
Age (years)			
mean ± s.d.	60 ± 11	59 ± 11	ns
Prior PTCA (%)	67	63	ns
Canadian Heart Class			ns
0	8	14	
I	3	5	
II	14	14	
III	36	24	
IV	39	43	

PTCA = percutaneous transluminal coronary angioplasty.

Table 2.
Baseline Lesion Characteristics

	Thrombosis	*No Thrombosis*	*p*
Eccentric (%)	47	55	ns
Calcification (%)	28	16	ns
Thrombus (%)	9	7	ns
Bend ≥ 45% (%)	11	14	ns
Vessel location (%)			ns
Left Main	0	1	
LAD	70	39	
Lcx	8	11	
RCA	22	49	
Lesion length (mm)	6.7 ± 5.0	7.6 ± 5.7	ns
Arterial diameter (mm)	2.9 ± 0.3	3.1 ± 0.5	0.01

LAD = left anterior descending artery; Lcx = left circumflex; RCA, right coronary artery.

vessel tortuosity, baseline percent-diameter stenosis, or lesion length. In patients who developed stent thrombosis, vessel size was noted to be smaller when compared to the group of patients who did not develop stent thrombosis (2.9 versus 3.1 mm).

Procedural Variables

Several procedural variables were noted to be associated with stent thrombosis. Figure 2 depicts the diameter stenosis at baseline, following conventional balloon angioplasty, and after stent placement. At baseline, there was no difference in the mean percent-diameter stenosis. However, following conventional balloon angioplasty, there was a difference. After balloon angioplasty, patients who developed stent thrombosis had a significantly larger residual diameter stenosis of 60% as compared to 48% for those without stent thrombosis. In contrast, there was no difference in the residual stenosis after stent placement between the two groups.

Figure 3 shows the two groups of patients with respect to the appearance of thrombus during the angioplasty procedure. Intraprocedural thrombus was noted in 28% of patients who developed stent thrombosis as compared to 9% who did not develop stent thrombosis ($P < 0.001$). The two groups were also compared with respect to the presence of intimal dissection. There was no difference between patients with and without stent thrombosis in the incidence of dissection following standard balloon angioplasty. In contrast, a residual dissection following stenting was twice as common in patients with stent thrombosis as compared to those without stent thrombosis (22% versus 11%) (Fig. 4). Therefore, while the presence of an intimal disruption prior to stent

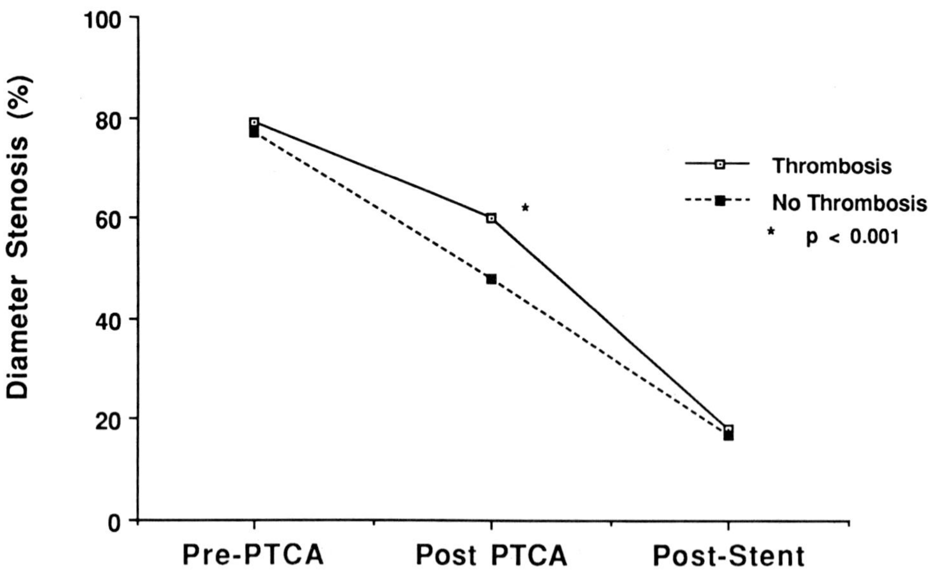

Figure 2: *Diameter stenosis at baseline, following conventional PTCA, and following stent implantation in patients with and without stent thrombosis. (PTCA = percutaneous transluminal coronary angioplasty).*

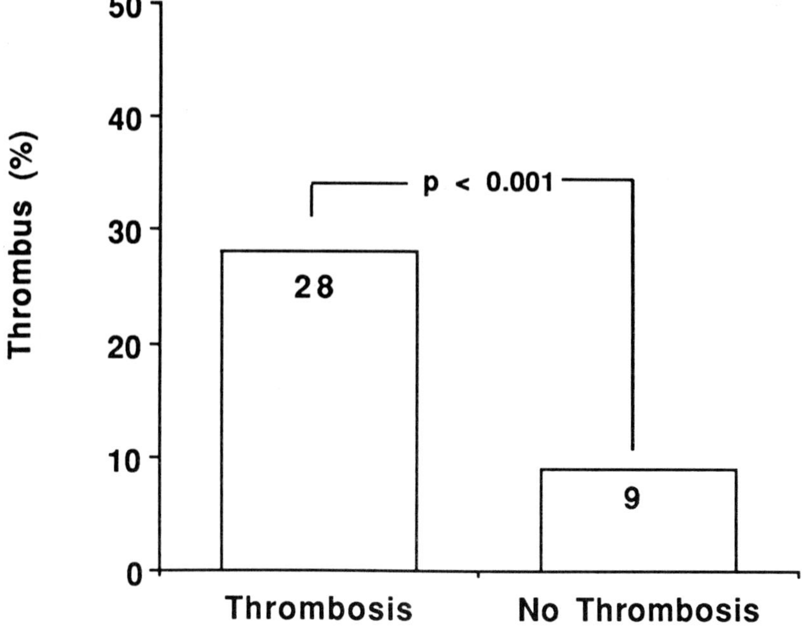

Figure 3: *A comparison of patients with and without stent thrombosis with respect to the procedural appearance of thrombus.*

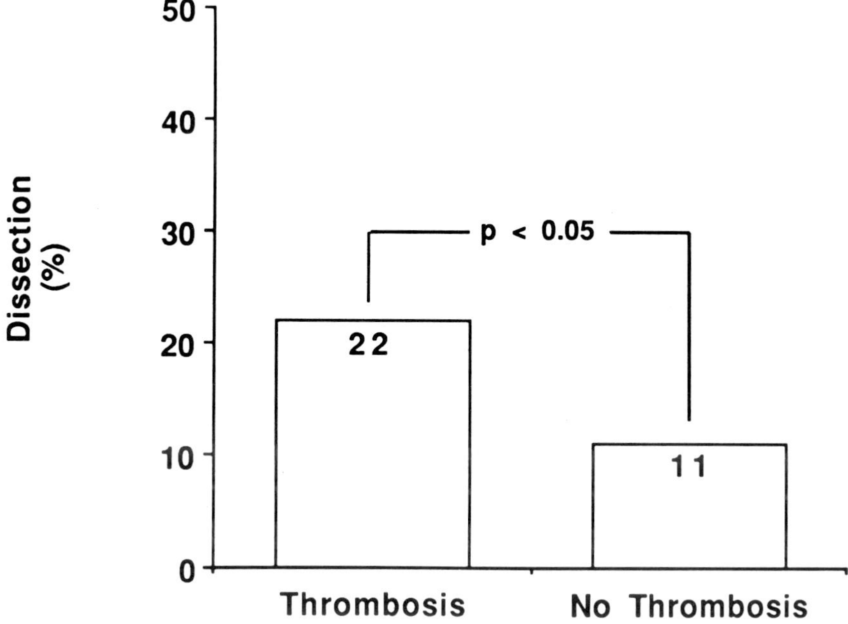

Figure 4: *A comparison of patients with and without stent thrombosis with respect to the presence of a dissection following stenting.*

placement was not predictive of stent thrombosis, the presence of a disruption after stent placement was a significant factor predictive of stent thrombosis.

Clinical Implications for Management

From this angiographic evaluation, we concluded that thrombosis following coronary stent placement is affected by several baseline angiographic and procedural factors. These include small-vessel size, significant residual stenosis after conventional balloon angioplasty, intraprocedural thrombus, and dissection following stent implantation. Intimal dissection due to balloon angioplasty which is successfully resolved by stenting is not associated with an increased risk of stent thrombosis. These results have important clinical implications for patient selection and for the management of patients after stent implantation. Important contraindications to stent placement include initial small-vessel size and a suboptimal angioplasty result associated with thrombus. In patients who have undergone coronary stenting, the persistence of a dissection or thrombus should be considered a marker for subsequent thrombotic occlusion. These patients should be monitored carefully, similar to the guidelines provided for patients receiving emergent stents (see Chapter 6).

Despite the ability to reestablish vessel patency with thrombolysis and repeat balloon angioplasty, stent thrombosis is associated with significant adverse clinical outcomes, including myocardial infarction and the need for emergency bypass surgery. In addition, most patients will require additional hospitalization for adjustment of the prothrombin time. Patients who have a thrombotic event after hospital discharge are at particular high risk for complications. This explains the high incidence of myocardial infarction (37%) and emergent coronary artery bypass surgery (37%) observed in patients with stent thrombosis.

Rapid recanalization of the artery is of obvious importance in reducing the complications of stent thrombosis. This can be achieved with intravenous lytic therapy, but hemorrhage from recent vascular catheterization sites presents a relative limitation of this approach. More often, patients are brought directly to the catheterization laboratory where repeat angioplasty is performed with the adjuvant use of intracoronary urokinase. In our experience, this may require a stiff guidewire to negotiate the large mass of thrombus. In patients who have persistent thrombus or dissection following repeat intervention, urgent coronary artery bypass surgery should be performed.

Illustrative Case

Figure 5 illustrates an example of a 40-year-old male who developed stent thrombosis. The baseline angiogram reveals a critical, eccentric stenosis of the proximal left anterior descending coronary artery (Fig. 5A). Following balloon angioplasty, a large, nonflow-limiting dissection can be seen at the site of the balloon dilation (Fig. 5B). Figure 5C shows the result following stent implantation. Despite improvement in the vessel lumen, a persistent nonobstructive linear flap distal to the stented segment can be seen (arrow). At 7 days following stent implantation, the patient developed ischemic pain with evidence of an acute anterior wall myocardial infarction on the electrocardiogram. Angiography at the time of presentation revealed a thrombotic occlusion of the stented vessel (Fig. 5D). The patient underwent repeat balloon dilation and infusion of intracoronary urokinase. Despite this treatment, persistent thrombus was noted, and the patient was sent for emergent coronary artery bypass surgery. Follow-up electrocardiograms revealed a non-Q-wave myocardial infarction.

This case emphasizes the significance of a suboptimal result following stent placement. In this example, the persistence of an intimal flap distal to the stent was a predisposing factor to stent thrombosis. An attempt to tack up such flaps should be made by additional prolonged balloon inflations or by deploying a second stent.

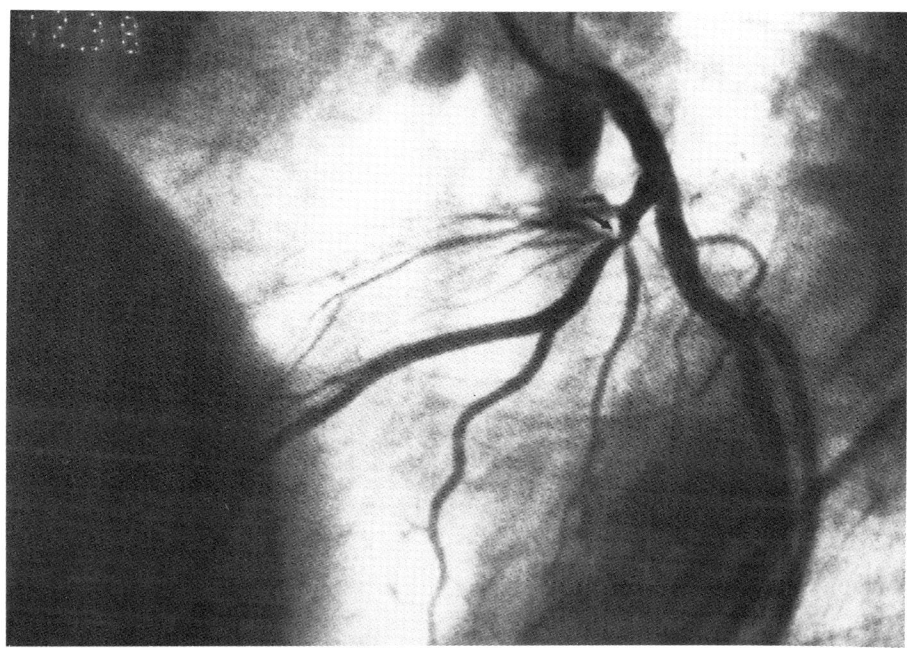

Figure 5A: *Baseline left coronary angiogram in the LAO projection. Note the critical, eccentric stenosis of the proximal left anterior descending coronary artery. (LAO = left anterior oblique).*

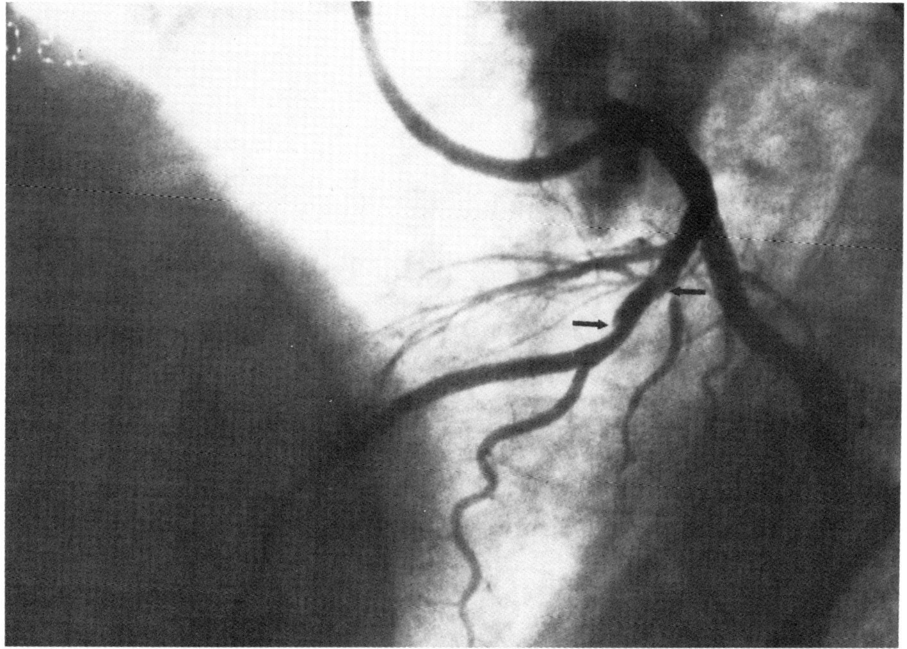

Figure 5B: *Result after conventional PTCA. A nonflow-limiting dissection can be seen at the site of balloon dilation. (PTCA = percutaneous transluminal coronary angioplasty).*

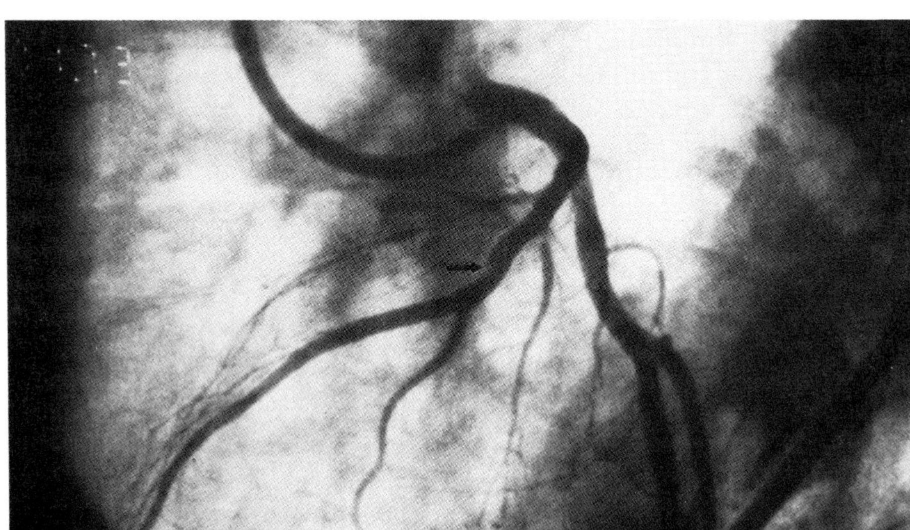

Figure 5C: *Result after placement of a single Palmaz-Schatz stent. Note the persistence of a nonobstructive, linear flap distal to the stented segment.*

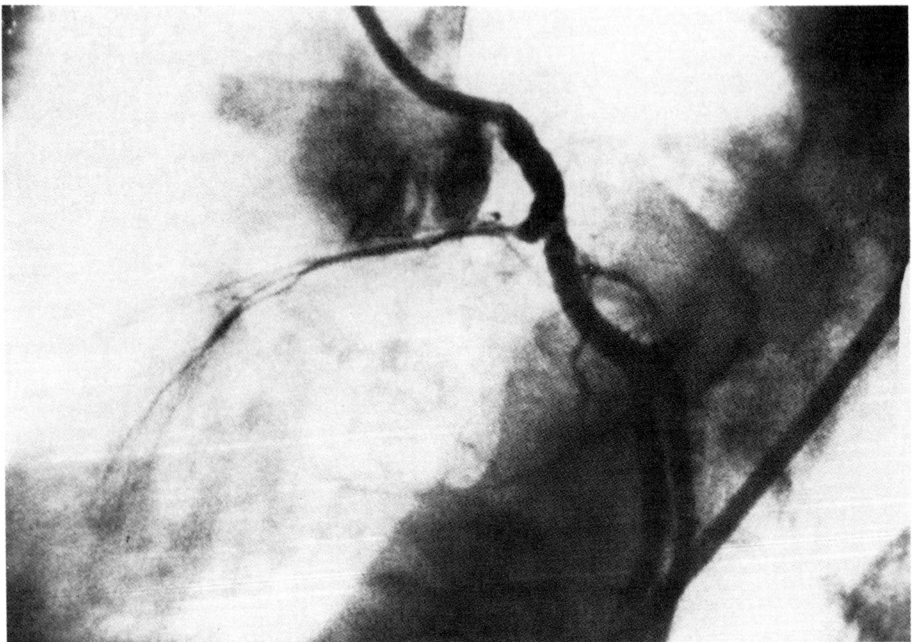

Figure 5D: *Emergent coronary angiogram at 7 days following stent implantation. There is a thrombotic occlusion of the stented vessel.*

Prevention of Stent Thrombosis

Despite the recognition of the need for vigorous anticoagulation in patients who have undergone stenting, stent thrombosis remains a major limitation. To this end, adjuvant technologies are being evaluated to help in the prevention of stent thrombosis. For example, coating of Palmaz-Schatz stents with synthetic polymers or heparin appears to reduce acute thrombus formation in experimental animals.[8] With the recognition that thrombogenicity of the stent is decreased as the stent surface is covered by regrowth of endothelium, preliminary studies evaluating the seeding of intravascular stents with genetically engineered endothelial cells have been performed.[9] In vitro studies have shown that intravascular stents can be coated with a layer of genetically engineered endothelial cells that can either be specifically labeled or made to secrete high levels of a therapeutic protein. Hopefully, an improvement in stent function will be realized with the localized delivery of anticoagulant, thrombolytic, or antiproliferative molecules.

REFERENCES

1. Serruys PW, Strauss BH, Beatt KJ, Bertrand ME, Puel J, Rickards AF, Meier B, Goy JJ, Vogt P, Kappenberger L, Sigwart U: Angiographic follow-up after placement of a single self-expanding coronary artery stent. *N Engl J Med* 1991; 324:13–17.
2. Macauder PJ, Agrawal SK, Roubin GS : The Gianturco-Roubin balloon-expandable intracoronary flexible coil stent. *J Invent Cardiol* 1991;3:85–94.
3. Buchwald A, Unterberg C, Werner G, Vath E, Kreuzer H, Wiegard V: Initial clinical results with the Wiktor stent: a new balloon-expandable coronary stent. *Clin Cardiol* 1991; 14:374–379.
4. Palmaz JC, Garcia 0, Kopp DT, Schatz RA, Tio FO, Ciarvino V: Balloon-expandable intra-arterial stents: effect of anticoagulation on thrombus formation. *Circulation* 1987; 76 (suppl IV):IV 45.
5. Schatz RA, Palmaz JC, Tio FO, Garcia F, Garcia O: Balloon expandable intracoronary stents in the adult dog: *Circulation* 1987;76:450–457.
6. Schatz RA, Baim DS, Leon M, Ellis SG, Goldberg S, Hirshfeld JW, Cleman MW, Cabin HS, Walker C, Stagg J, Buchbinder M, Teirstein PS, Topol EJ, Savage M, Perez JA, Curry RC, Whitworth H, Sousa JE, Tio FO, Almagor Y, Ponder R, Penn IM, Leonard B, Levine SL, Fish DR, Palmaz JC: Clinical experience with the Palmaz-Schatz coronary stent: initial results of a multicenter study. *Circulation* 1991;83: 148–161.
7. Fischman DL, Savage MP, Leon MB, Hirshfeld JW, Cleman MW, Teirstein P, Goldberg S: Angiographic predictors of subacute thrombosis following coronary artery stenting. *Circulation* 1991; 84(suppl)II:II 588.
8. Bailey SR, Guy DM, Garcia BJ, Paige S, Palmaz J, Miller DD: Polymer coating of Palmaz-Schatz stent attenuates vascular spasm after stent placement. *Circulation* 1990; 82(suppl III):III 541.
9. Dicheck DA, Neville RF, Zwiebel JA, Freeman SM, Leon MB, Anderson WF: Seeding of intravascular stents with genetically engineered endothelial cells. *Circulation* 1989;80:1347–1353.

CHAPTER 9

Peripheral Vascular Complications of Coronary Endovascular Stent Placement

Michael A. Golden
Stephen W. Downing

This chapter will discuss the peripheral vascular complications of coronary endovascular stent placement. Because of the paucity of reports on stenting procedures, we will also include in our discussion information derived from the described complications of other invasive percutaneous coronary procedures which may be applicable to stent placement. Each complication will be discussed below in terms of incidence, risk factors, possible prevention, and management. The role of prompt surgical consultation in cases of suspected hemorrhage or ischemia of the limb or gut cannot be overemphasized, as delays in therapy are associated with significant morbidity and mortality.

Incidence of Vascular Complications

The incidence of peripheral vascular complications from percutaneous diagnostic cardiac catheterizations and percutaneous transluminal coronary angioplasty (PTCA) has been well documented, and is between 0.2% and 2%[1–13] (see Tables 1 and 2). Furthermore, in a prospective study, Kresowik et al[1] evaluated every femoral artery puncture site with color-flow duplex scanning, and detected vascular complications in 9% of patients. One-third of these injuries eventually required operative correction. While the high sensitivity of this technique may overestimate the incidence of "clinically significant" lesions, it demonstrates that more vascular trauma occurs than is evident on routine postprocedural physical examination.

The complications most commonly noted are: bleeding or massive hematoma or both, pseudoaneurysm, peripheral ischemia, arteriovenous fistulae,

From: Herrmann HC, Hirshfeld JW, eds. *Clinical Use of the Palmaz-Schatz Intracoronary Stent.* Futura Publishing Company, Inc., Mount Kisco, NY, © 1993.

Table 1.
Complication Data from Reports of Diagnostic Catheterization or Percutaneous Transluminal Coronary Angioplasty Procedures

				Complication Rates (%)				
					Percentage due to:			
Reference	*Type*	*n*	*Route*	*Overall*	*Ischemia*	*Pseudo Ay*	*Hemorrhage*	*AVF*
Kresowik, 1991[1]	Dx/PTCA	144	Fem	9.0*	8	62		23
Babu, 1989[2]	Dx/PTCA	5,850	Fem	0.6	7	28	57	7
	Dx/PTCA	10,500	Brach	0.2	83	7	10	0
Kaufman, 1989[3]	Dx	2,904	Fem	1.2	20	3	57	
	PTCA	644	Fem	0.9	16	50	16	
Johnson, 1989[4]	Dx/PTCA	148,262	Fem	0.3				
	Dx/PTCA	67,575	Brach	1.0				
Oweida, 1990[5]	PTCA	4,988	Fem	1.1	11	64	11	14
Bredlau, 1985[6]	PTCA	3,500	Fem	0.7				
Dorros, 1983[7]	PTCA	1,500	Fem/Brach	1.5	55	10	30	5

* prospective evaluation with color-flow duplex scanning
Diagnostic (dx); percutaneous transluminal coronary angioplasty (PTCA); femoral (fem); brachial (brach); pseudoaneurysm pseudo (Ay); arteriovenous fistuale (AVF).

Table 2.
Complication Data from Reports Including Complex Cardiologic Percutaneous Interventions

				Complication Rates (%)				
					Percentage due to:			
Reference	*Type*	*n*	*Route*	*Overall*	*Ischemia*	*Pseudo Ay*	*Hemorrhage*	*AVF*
Skillman, 1988[8]	Dx	5,431	Fem	0.6	10	64	13	13
	PTCA	1,747	Fem	1.0	6	59	6	29
	PBV	155	Fem	5.2	25	25	38	12
	IABP	209	Fem	11.5	85	10	5	
Muller, 1992[9]	Dx	1,519	Fem	0.6				
	PTCA	698	Fem	2.6				
	Other	183	Fem	6.0				
Safian, 1990[10]	DCA	67	Fem	3.0				
Wyman, 1988[11]	All	2,741	Fem	1.9	21	57	9	13
	Dx	1,609	Fem	1.6				
	PTCA	933	Fem	1.5				
	PBV	199	Fem	7.5				
Schatz, 1991[12]	Stent	226	Fem	8.4	0	16	47	
Roubin, 1992[13]	Stent	115	Fem	7.8	0	78	11	11

Diagnostic (dx), percutaneous transluminal coronary angioplasty (PTCA), femoral (fem), pseudoaneurysm (pseudo Ay), arteriovenous fistuale (AVF), percutaneous balloon valvuloplasty (PBV), directional coronary atherectomy (DCA), intra-aortic balloon pump (IABP).

peripheral emboli, and femoral neuralgia. Factors that appear to increase the incidence of periprocedural vascular complications include: advanced age,[5,9] small-vessel size, or gender (with females having generally smaller vessels),[5,8] peripheral vascular disease,[8,9] the use of sheaths larger than 8F,[3,9] and the periprocedural use of heparin or fibrinolytic agents.[1,5,8,9] In general, there is no difference in the overall incidence of complications between femoral and brachial access sites when comparing the rates for the preferred technique of each reporting institution. However, the femoral route is more likely to have bleeding, and the brachial route to have ischemic complications.[2]

Because complex percutaneous coronary interventional procedures such as stent placement and atherectomy often require larger sheaths, multiple catheter exchanges, and commit the patient to a course of anticoagulation, an increased incidence of peripheral vascular complications would be expected. This prediction has been borne out in several series as summarized in Table 2,[8–13] where the complication rate for complex interventional procedures greatly exceeded the 1% rate expected for diagnostic procedures. In complex interventional cases, there was a tendency toward more bleeding and less ischemic complications, which likely reflects the extensive use of anticoagulation in these patients. Another complication unique to stent placement is peripheral stent embolization. In one large, multicenter series, this was reported to occur in 2.5% of placement attempts.[12] While none of these patients developed clinical sequelae, this represents a potentially significant peripheral vascular risk. The more recent development of a stent-delivery sheath (see Chapter 2) should further reduce the importance of this particular complication.

Preprocedure Peripheral Vascular History

The preprocedure peripheral vascular history is obviously important in choosing sites for catheterization, and is critical for evaluating the patient once a problem has occurred. Careful attention should be paid to a history of claudication, rest pain, poorly healing leg wounds, and prior invasive procedures or surgery. The site of claudication is helpful in differentiating aortoiliac (buttock and thigh claudication) from superficial femoral artery disease (calf claudication). All peripheral pulses should be carefully documented, and occlusion pressures recorded for any vessel that has only a Doppler signal.

Hemorrhage

A small hematoma after a catheterization is common, but a significant bleed can be dangerous and, frequently, difficult to diagnose early.[5] Patients undergoing invasive cardiac procedures have significant cardiac diseases including ischemia, arrhythmias, or cardiac failure, which may obscure the cause of hypotension. Postprocedural bleeding should be suspected whenever there is significant hypotension, with or without tachycardia. Measurement of central venous pressures may be helpful. The hemoglobin and hematocrit are not reliable indicators of a bleed as they do not change acutely.

The patterns of hematoma spread from femoral catheterization are well described[14] (Fig. 1), and include the deep fascial planes into the thigh, along the retroperitoneum into the pelvis, along the abdominal wall, and into the perineum (often with impressive scrotal or labial hematomas). It is possible to hemorrhage several liters of blood in these regions without any external signs. As seen in Figure 2, computed axial tomography may reveal an extensive retroperitoneal hematoma not evident on physical examination. Intraperitoneal bleeding may occur with a puncture above the inguinal ligament.

Factors that put the patient at risk for hemorrhage include excessively high or low punctures (where the vessel cannot be compressed against the femoral head), the use of anticoagulants and large sheaths, through-and-through puncture of the artery, a puncture on the medial or lateral side of the artery (where effective compression is difficult to obtain), and puncture of the artery on the medial or lateral aspect with laceration of a side branch.[3,5,8,15] Inadequate postprocedure manual groin compression has also been implicated.[15] Once a large hematoma has formed, it is difficult to reliably stop bleeding from the puncture site.

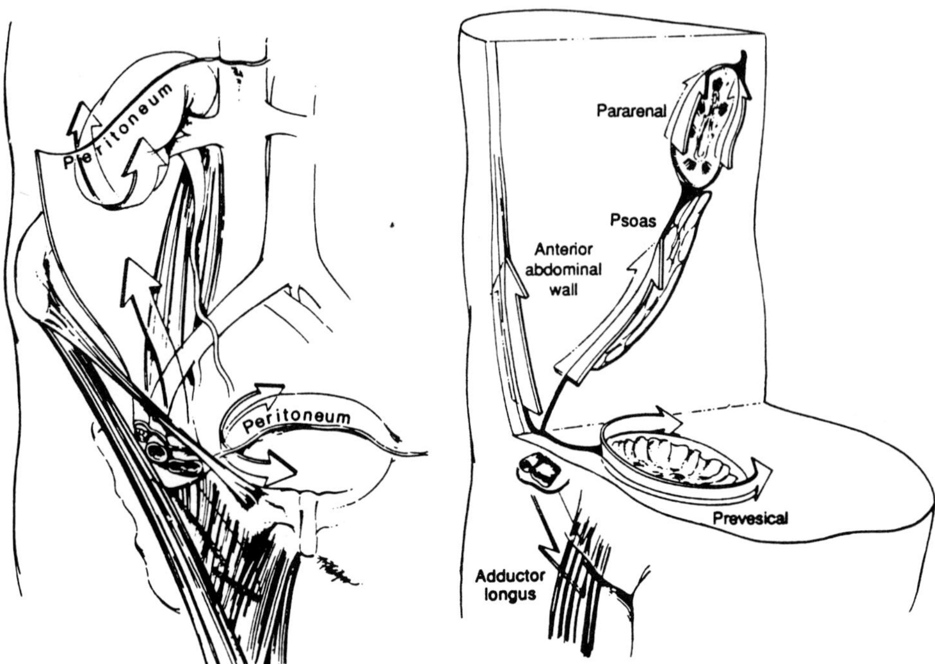

Figure 1: *These diagrams reveal the patterns of extension of angiographically related retroperitoneal hematomas. (From,[14] with permission).*

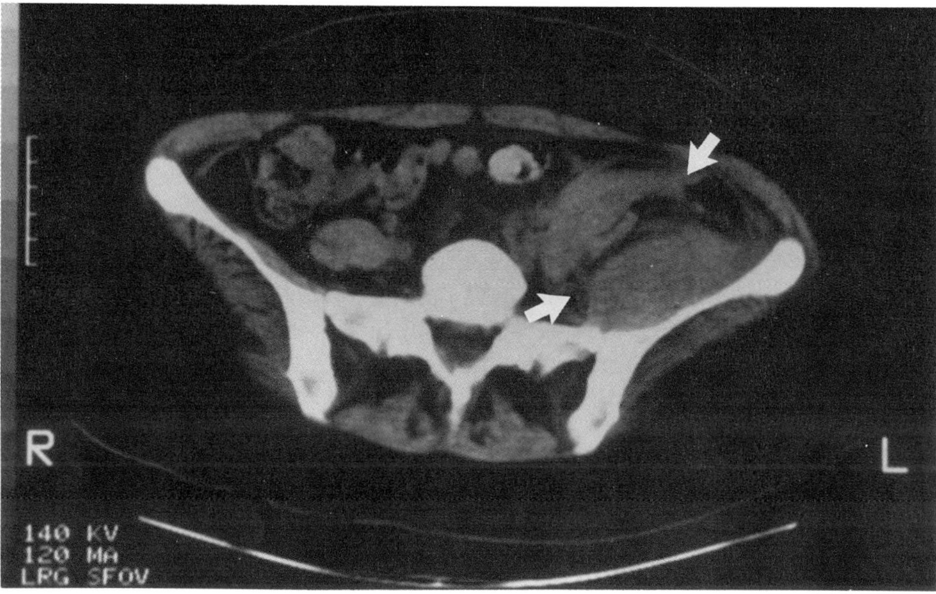

Figure 2: *The appearance on CT scan of a large left retroperitoneal hematoma (arrows) tracking from the left femoral artery catheterization site, cephalad along the psoas muscle into the pelvis and retroperitoneum.*

The first line of therapy should be volume expansion, with the placement of large peripheral intravenous lines (16 gauge or larger). A large venous introducer (i.e., 8F) is an excellent volume line. Blood should be crossmatched and available. Several liters of crystalloid may be required acutely, and the urine output via Foley catheter is a generally reliable guide to the adequacy of the resuscitation. Physicians are often reluctant to give a patient with cardiac disease large amounts of volume, but this is often what is indicated. If possible, any anticoagulation should be reversed or at the least decreased.

Prompt surgical repair is indicated for ongoing bleeding or hypotension, and any bleed that requires significant transfusion. According to Kaufman, the development of "hypotension, lower quadrant abdominal mass or femoral neuropathy is ominous in the presence of a groin hematoma," and indicates the need for exploration.[3] Imaging studies are generally not helpful and only delay appropriate therapy.

Depending on the site of injury, the vessel may be approached from the groin, in the pelvic retroperitoneum via a suprainguinal "transplant incision," or through the abdomen. Proximal and distal control are attained, and the rent oversewn. Broadly damaged segments may require prosthetic grafting or vein patching. General anesthesia is preferred in case the iliac artery or aorta needs to be approached in the pelvis or abdomen.

Pseudoaneurysm

A pseudoaneurysm is an aneurysm lacking all three layers of the arterial wall (intima, media, and adventitia). Practically speaking, it is an advanced hematoma with a liquefied center that is still in communication with the arterial flow via the arterial wall puncture site. Its expansion is confined by the local connective tissue, which with time will form a fibrous layer around it.

Differentiating a pseudoaneurysm from a hematoma with a transmitted pulse can be difficult. A pseudoaneurysm should have radially pulsatile expansion, whereas a hematoma should only have a palpable pulsation from posterior to anterior. The presence or absence of a bruit is not specific. The current gold standard for diagnosis is color-flow duplex scanning performed by someone experienced in peripheral vascular imaging.[16,17] This will show swirling blood flow in the pseudoaneurysm cavity, and can delineate where the arterial anatomy has been injured Fig. 3. The anatomical information provided by duplex scanning is helpful if surgical repair is needed, and can, on occasion, be used therapeutically (see below). Other injuries should also be sought such as neuralgia from femoral nerve compression by the pseudoaneurysm,[18] arteriovenous fistula, which occasionally coexists with pseudoaneurysms,[1] and signs of peripheral ischemia from concurrent intimal flaps or distal emboli.

Pseudoaneurysms represent 30% to 60% of all vascular complications (Tables 1 and 2). Risk factors are similar to those for bleeding, and include the use of heparin, inadequate compression after sheath removal, the use of large sheaths, and an arterial puncture located in an area that is not easily compressible.[1,3,16,17] The natural history of catheter-induced pseudoaneurysms is not known.[1,16,17,18,19] Older surgical dogma stated that all pseudoaneurysms should be repaired upon detection, due to the risks of skin necrosis and aneurysm rupture. In one series, two out of three patients with ruptured pseudoaneurysms died.[17] However, much of the traditional surgical approach was based on experience with postoperative anastomotic pseudoaneurysms,[1,18] which are often either technical or infectious in nature, and likely behave differently than catheter-induced pseudoaneurysms. There have been incidental reports of spontaneous thrombosis of small pseudoaneurysms,[17,19] and in one series that prospectively followed asymptomatic pseudoaneurysms of less than 3.5 cm, 7/7 pseudoaneurysms thrombosed by 4 weeks.[1] In another study, 5/6 thrombosed over a mean of 18 days.[16]

Currently, the first line of therapy should be direct compression of the neck of the pseudoaneurysm under ultrasound guidance. Fellmeth et al[20] reported successful closure of 27 of 29 femoral artery pseudoaneurysms with no long-term complications. Our experience at the Hospital of the University of Pennsylvania has not been as favorable, but the technique is promising. Analgesia

Color Figure 3 appears on p. 150A.

can be a problem during compression, thereby limiting its effectiveness, as firm pressure often needs to be placed on a tender groin for up to 30 minutes. If this fails, we recommend conservatively following a reliable patient with an asymptomatic pseudoaneurysm, measuring less than 3 cm in diameter, and having no signs of expansion. The patient should have a repeat scan within the first 5 to 7 days, then as indicated clinically until pseudoaneurysm thrombosis occurs. The effect of prolonged anticoagulation on this process is not known, but might prompt earlier surgical intervention. Large, expanding or symptomatic aneurysms should be operated on as soon as the patient's condition will tolerate.

Surgical repair can be performed under local anesthesia, though regional or general is preferred. The vessel is controlled proximally and distally if possible, and then the pseudoaneurysm cavity is entered. Usually, there is a small hole in the artery that requires one or two sutures for repair, and the long-term results are excellent.[5,18] Potential operative complications include arterial thromboembolism, bleeding, or incidental venous injury, which would require intraoperative correction. Other potential complications include infection, nerve injury, and the development of a lymphocele. Most nerve injuries are transient and can be treated expectantly. A lymphocele is a benign lymphatic collection that can be differentiated from an abscess by the minimal erythema, and lack of significant tenderness. These should be treated with frequent sterile-needle aspirations until they resolve.

Arteriovenous Fistula

Arteriovenous fistulae (AVF) represent about 5% to 30% of all the vascular complications of catheterization procedures. They appear to occur no more commonly in complex than in diagnostic procedures (Tables 1 and 2). Factors that increase the risk of fistula formation include double-wall puncture (or through-and-through puncture) of the femoral artery, punctures below the common femoral artery (superficial femoral or profunda femoral vessels), and simultaneous instrumentation of artery and vein.[1,5,8,21] Figure 4 demonstrates that the femoral vein is essentially behind the superficial femoral artery, making fistula formation more likely with poor technique. A bruit should raise the suspicion of fistula formation, but many other conditions can produce this, including preexisting peripheral vascular disease, traumatic vessel irregularities, and pseudoaneurysm. The classical findings on physical examination are a continuous bruit and a palpable thrill.[5] Late symptoms of AVF include angina, congestive heart failure, and claudication or leg ischemia (via a "steal" phenomenon).[8,21]

Suspicious areas should be evaluated with duplex scanning. Figure 5 reveals the color-flow duplex appearance of an AVF with constant fistula flow throughout the cardiac cycle. Although many surgeons will request angiography prior to undertaking repair, this should not be a primary diagnostic modality. The present treatment is surgical repair,[1,21] though ultrasound-guided

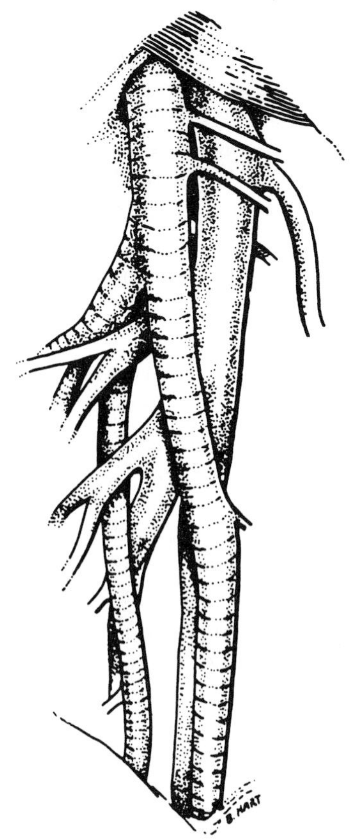

Figure 4: *The close spatial relationship between the femoral arterial vessels and venous vessels results in the not infrequent occurrence of arteriovenous fistula formation after puncture. Note that the femoral vein passes directly behind the superficial femoral artery. (Adapted from,[21] with permission).*

Color Figure 5 appears on p. 150A.

compression may be applicable to these lesions as well.[20] The operation is straightforward, with good results and a minimal complication rate. While spontaneous resolution has been reported,[17] most series report persistence of the AVF over time,[1,8] with the potential for enlargement and aneurysmal degeneration. Repair can be done electively if there are no cardiac or peripheral vascular symptoms.[1,17]

Limb Ischemia

Limb ischemia can be the most morbid complication of percutaneous cardiac procedures. This represents anywhere between 7% and 25% of all vascular complications using the femoral approach, and up to 80% from the brachial. With the common use of anticoagulation, it is likely that ischemia will be less common with stent placement. Indeed, neither Schatz[12] nor Herrmann[22] had occurrences of limb ischemia in their series.

The brachial approach, because of vessel size, is less suitable for most complex catheterization procedures, but merits brief discussion. In comparison to the femoral artery, the brachial artery has less bleeding complications and more ischemic complications.[2,4] The loss of a previously palpable pulse should prompt vascular surgical consultation. A Doppler signal at the wrist with a viable hand does not exclude the presence of major artery thrombosis. Two major complications can develop; the first is long-term limb dysfunction with hand claudication. Machleder et al reported a 37% incidence of severe disability in follow-up of patients who had lost their radial pulse.[23] The second is progression of the thrombosis. A radial artery Doppler signal may be due to flow from the ulnar artery via the palmar arch. When the brachial artery is thrombosed, collaterals will sustain the hand initially, but without anticoagulation, the thrombus may propagate. Eventually, higher collaterals such as the superior ulnar and the deep brachial may occlude and render the limb critically ischemic. Repair usually requires resection and end-to-end anastomosis.[2] Vein-patch angioplasty may be required for brachial artery reconstruction in areas involved with dissection or intimal flaps.

Lower limb ischemia can result from vessel thrombosis, arterial dissection, the development of intimal flaps, or from embolization of clot or plaque. Risk factors include peripheral vascular disease and inadvertent puncture of the superficial femoral or profunda femoral arteries (which are smaller in diameter compared to the common femoral artery). Other risk factors include large sheath size, and lack of periprocedural anticoagulation.[3,8,9,15,17] The wires used during percutaneous vascular procedures are thrombogenic, and long periods with indwelling wires or catheters can lead to thrombosis and embolization.[3,15] Excessive compression of the femoral vessels can also lead to thrombosis. The diagnosis can usually be made clinically with the characteristic findings of a cool limb with pain, pallor, pulselessness, paralysis, or paresthesias. A decrease in pulses with a sheath in place is of concern, but this is often a function of the sheath's presence alone, and is not grounds for action without clinical signs of limb ischemia.[8] The loss of motor function is a grave sign. Angiography is usually not necessary, since delays in diagnosis and therapy correlate with morbidity and mortality.[2]

For most occlusions, the surgical treatment of choice is embolectomy and catheter thrombectomy. The vessel is opened at the puncture site and a balloon catheter is passed proximally and distally to remove all thrombus. Contributing injuries such as intimal flaps or large atherosclerotic plaques are also repaired. Severely diseased vessels frequently require vein-patch angioplasty[8] (35% in one series[2]). The revascularization of ischemic muscle can cause a reperfusion injury, with the subsequent release of potassium and myoglobin, and the development of significant muscular edema. Lower-leg fasciotomy may be indicated to prevent compartment syndrome. The results of surgical therapy are usually good,[5,17] but perioperative complication rates of up to 20% have been reported.[8] Delayed repair can have a morbidity rate of nearly 30%,[2] with a high rate of limb loss and ischemic neuropathy.[2,8]

The optimal therapy for less severe distal emboli is controversial. The loss of one vessel in the lower leg with good flow and collateral circulation from another may be followed conservatively. Unfortunately, there are little data on the long-term morbidity of this approach. Small distal atheromatous emboli may cause spotting on the bottom of the foot, resulting in the so-called "trash foot." If there is no significant tissue loss or suprainfection, these can also be watched expectantly. Cholesterol embolization may occur, and is, on occasion, clinically significant.[15] These emboli can shower the lower extremities, kidneys, bowel, and pancreas. This may be associated with fever and a livedo reticularis pattern in the skin of the lower extremities and genitalia.[15,24] The mortality of this rare entity can be up to 67%.[25]

Mesenteric Ischemia

Mesenteric ischemia is a rare but exceptionally devastating complication occurring in less than 1% of all procedures.[5] The mortality rate is greater than 85%. The most common mechanism is embolization of atherosclerotic debris from aortic plaque. The material becomes lodged in the superior mesenteric artery and causes end-organ ischemia. Aortic dissection is another less common possible etiology. The classic presentation is one of severe abdominal pain out of proportion to physical examination, often accompanied by bowel evacuation. The patient may begin to complain of abdominal pain on the cardiac catheterization table. There is no predictive laboratory examination (including white blood cell count, pH, amylase, and phosphate). Immediate angiographic examination of the mesenteric arterial anatomy is warranted followed, without delay, by surgical exploration and restoration of mesenteric arterial blood flow. Early surgical consultation is recommended whenever the diagnosis is suspected.

Infection

Infection is a rare complication of catheterization and can present as a septicemia, pseudoaneurysm, or infected hematoma.[26,27] Distal septic emboli and regional septic arthritis or osteomyelitis also have been reported.[26] Frazee and Flaherty noted that all of their cases were associated with repeat PTCA or repeat puncture at a site of prior PTCA.[27] McCready noted similar observations, with all of their cases involving repeat ipsilateral puncture or sheaths left in place for 1 to 5 days.[26] The purported mechanism is colonization of the catheter or its tract with skin flora. In all reported cases, the infecting organism was *Staphylococcus aureus*. This is a morbid occurrence, with 2/9 of McCready's patients dying.

The risk of infectious complications in stenting is not known, but Herrmann[22] reported the occurrence of a groin abscess in their series of patients receiving emergent stents. It is likely that with anticoagulation-associated hematomas, repeat puncture, and prolonged sheath retention, this complication will be observed with increased frequency. The therapy should be antibiotics directed against skin flora, and prompt surgical evacuation of any collections. Complex vascular reconstruction may be needed.[26] Computer scanning, searching for occult-infected retroperitoneal hematomas should be considered in any patient with unexplained sepsis. Large occult collections have been reported.[14,26] prophylactic antibiotics are currently recommended for stent procedures.

Neuralgia

Several series have reported femoral neuralgia as a "co-complication" of catheterization, often seen with large hematomas or pseudoaneurysms. The neuralgia results from compression or irritation of the two anterior cutaneous branches of the femoral nerve[28] (see Fig. 6). This usually presents as groin

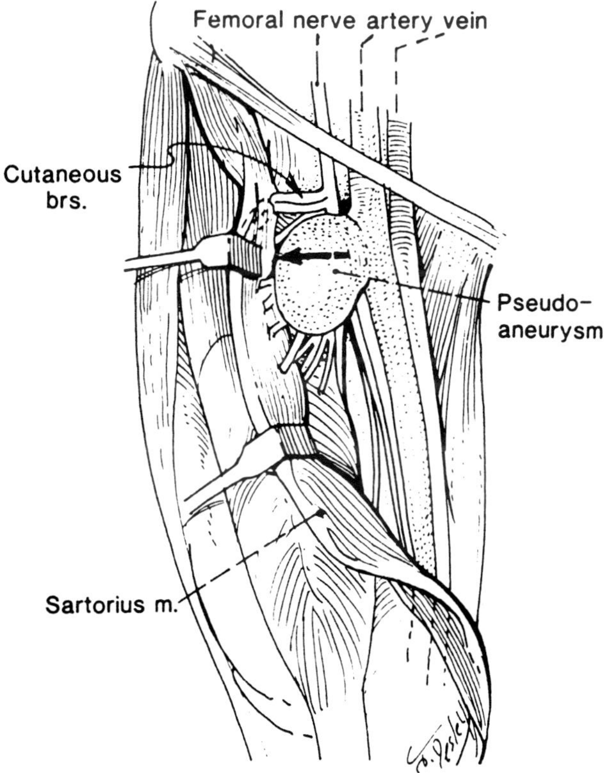

Figure 6: *The illustration demonstrates the close anatomical relationship of a femoral pseudoaneurysm and the anterior cutaneous branches of the femoral nerve, which may result in femoral neuralgias after catheterization. (From,[28] with permission).*

pain, with or without anteromedial thigh pain, and is often associated with hyperesthesias. This complication has been reported in up to one-third of patients requiring surgery for vascular complications.[28,29] In addition to surgical correction of the inciting entity, neuralgia should be treated symptomatically with nonsteroidal anti-inflammatory medications. Tricyclic antidepressants and femoral nerve block also have been reported to be helpful.[28]

Device Embolization

Embolism of both the femoral sheath[30] and the coronary stent device[3] have been reported. Embolized sheaths should be recovered after they have been radiographically localized. The much smaller stents are not easily appreciated on radiography. In the Schatz series, despite the 3% rate of stent embolization, there were no reported incidences of vascular compromise.[12] The recommendation at this point would be an attempted localization of embolized stents, followed by close observation of the affected site for signs of vascular compromise. It is possible that late complications could develop, however, the true long-term risk is not known. It is likely that increased experience and improved delivery systems will make device embolization less common.

Summary

Coronary endovascular stent placement is associated with a low, but significant incidence of peripheral vascular complications. These vary from minor hematomas to lethal hemorrhagic or ischemic problems. Meticulous technique, a full understanding of the potential associated complications, and early detection and treatment may allow the incidence of vascular complications to be reduced and their clinical sequelae minimized.

REFERENCES

1. Kresowik TF, Khoury MD, Miller BV, Winniford MD, Shamma AR, Sharp WJ, Blecha MB, Corson JD: A prospective study of the incidence and natural history of femoral vascular complications after percutaneous transluminal coronary angioplasty. *J Vas Surg* 1991; 13:328–336.
2. Babu SC, Piccorelli GO, Shah PM, Stein JH, Clauss RH: Incidence and results of arterial complications among 16,350 patients undergoing cardiac catheterization. *J Vas Surg* 1989; 10:113–116.
3. Kaufman J, Moglia R, Lacy C, Dinerstein C, Moreyra A: Peripheral vascular complications from percutaneous transluminal coronary angioplasty: a comparison with transfemoral cardiac catheterization. *Am J Med Sci* 1989; 297:22–25.
4. Johnson LW, Lozner EC, Johnson S, Krone R, Pichard AD, Vetrovec GW, Noto TJ, and the Registry Committee of the Society for Cardiac Angiography and Interventions: Coronary angiography 1984–1987: a report of the registry of the Society for Cardiac Angiography and Interventions. *Cathet Cardiovasc Diagn* 1989; 17:5–10.
5. Oweida SW, Roubin GS, Smith RB III, Salam AA: Postcatheterization vascular

complications associated with percutaneous transluminal coronary angioplasty. *J Vas Surg* 1990; 12:310–315.

6. Bredlau CE, Roubin GS, Leimgruber PP, Douglas JS Jr, King SB III, Gruentzig AR: In-hospital morbidity and mortality in patients undergoing elective coronary angioplasty. *Circulation* 1985; 72:1044–1052.
7. Dorros G, Cowley MJ, Simpson J, Bentivoglio LG, Block PC, Bourassa M, Detre K, Gosselin AJ, Gruntzig AR, Kelsey SF, Kent KM, Mock MB, Mullin SM, Myler RK, Passamani ER, Stertzer SH, Williams DO: Percutaneous transluminal coronary angioplasty: report of complications from the National Heart, Lung, and Blood Institute PTCA Registry. *Circulation* 1983; 67:723–730.
8. Skillman JJ, Kim D, Baim DS: Vascular complications of percutaneous femoral cardiac interventions. *Arch Surg* 1988; 123:1207–1212.
9. Muller DWM, Shamir KJ, Ellis SG, Topol EJ: Peripheral vascular complications after conventional and complex percutaneous coronary interventional procedures. *Am J Cardiol* 1992; 69:63–68.
10. Safian RD, Gelbfish JS, Erny RE, Schnitt SJ, Schmidt DA, Baim DS: Coronary atherectomy: clinical, angiographic, and histological findings and observations regarding potential mechanisms. *Circulation* 1990; 82:69–79.
11. Wyman RM, Safian RD, Portway V, Skillman JJ, McKay RG, Baim DS: Current complications of diagnostic and therapeutic cardiac catheterization. *J Am Coll Cardiol* 1988; 12:1400–1406.
12. Schatz RA, Baim DS, Leon M, Ellis SG, Goldberg S, Hirshfeld JW, Cleman MW, Cabin HS, Walker C, Stagg J, Buchbinder M, Tierstein PS, Topol EJ, Savage M, Perez JA, Curry RC, Whitworth H, Sousa JE, Tio FO, Almagor Y, Ponder R, Penn IM, Leonard B, Levine SL, Fish RD, Palmaz JC: Clinical experience with the Palmaz-Schatz coronary stent: initial results of a multicenter study. *Circulation* 1991; 83:148–161.
13. Roubin GS, Cannon AD, Agrawal SK, Macander PJ, Dean LS, Baxley WA, Breland J: Intracoronary stenting for acute and threatened closure complicating percutaneous transluminal coronary angioplasty. *Circulation* 1992; 85:916–927.
14. Trerotola SO, Kuhlman JE, Fishman EK: Bleeding complications of femoral catheterization: CT evaluation. *Radiology* 1990; 174:37–40.
15. Kim D, Orron DE: Techniques and complications of angiography. In: Kim D, Orron DE, eds. *Peripheral Vascular Imaging and Intervention.* St. Louis: Mosby Year Book; 1990:83–109.
16. Johns JP, Pupa LE Jr, Bailey SR: Spontaneous thrombosis of iatrogenic femoral artery pseudoaneurysms: documentation with color Doppler and two-dimensional ultrasonography. *J Vas Surg* 1991; 14:24–29.
17. McCann RL, Schwartz LB, Pieper KS: Vascular complications of cardiac catheterization. *J Vas Surg* 1991; 14:375–381.
18. Roberts SR, Main D, Pinkerton J: Surgical therapy of femoral artery pseudoaneurysm after angiography. *Am J Surg* 1987; 154:676–680.
19. Kotval PS, Khoury A, Shah PM, Babu SC: Doppler sonographic demonstration of the progressive spontaneous thrombosis of pseudoaneurysms. *J Ultrasound Med* 1990; 9:185–190.
20. Fellmeth BD, Roberts AC, Bookstein JJ, Freischlag JA, Forsythe JR, Buckner NK, Hye RJ: Postangiographic femoral artery injuries: nonsurgical repair with US-guided compression. *Radiology* 1991; 178:671–675.
21. Lamar R, Berg R, Rama K: Femoral arteriovenous fistula as a complication of percutaneous transluminal coronary angioplasty: a report of five cases. *Am Surg* 1990; 56:702–706.
22. Herrmann HC, Buchbinder M, Clemen MW, Fischman D, Goldberg S, Leon MB, Schatz RA, Tierstein P, Walker CM, Hirshfeld JW Jr: Emergent use of balloon-expandable coronary artery stenting for failed PTCA. *Circulation* 1992; 86: 812–819.

23. Machleder HI, Sweeney JP, Barker WF: Pulseless arm after brachial-artery catheterisation. *Lancet* 1972; 1:407–409.
24. Rosansky SJ: Multiple cholesterol emboli syndrome after angiography. *AJR* 1984; 143:683.
25. Gaines PA, Kennedy A, Moorhead P, Cumberland DC, Welsh CL, Rutley MS: Cholesterol embolisation: a lethal complication of vascular catheterisation. *Lancet* 1988; 19:168.
26. McCready RA, Siderys H, Pittman JN, Herod GT, Halbrook HG, Fehrenbacher JW, Beckman DJ, Hormuth DA: Septic complications after cardiac catheterization and percutaneous transluminal coronary angioplasty. *J Vas Surg* 1991; 14: 170–174.
27. Frazee BW, Flaherty JP: Septic endarteritis of the femoral artery following angioplasty. *Rev Infect Dis* 1991; 13:620–623.
28. Hallett JW Jr, Wolk SW, Cherry KJ Jr, Gloviczki P, Pairolero PC: The femoral neuralgia syndrome after arterial catheter trauma. *J Vas Surg* 1990; 11:702–706.
29. Cohen JR, Sardari F, Glener L, Peralo J, Grunwald A, Friedman G, Koss J, Nwasokwa O, Bodenheimer M: Complications of diagnostic cardiac catheterization requiring surgical intervention. *Am J Cardiol* 1991; 67:787–788.
30. Messina LM, Brothers TE, Wakefield TW, Zelenock GB, Lindenauer SM, Greenfield LJ, Jacobs LA, Fellows EP, Grube SV, Stanley JC: Clinical characteristics and surgical management of vascular complications in patients undergoing cardiac catheterization: interventional versus diagnostic procedures. *J Vas Surg* 1991; 13: 593–600.

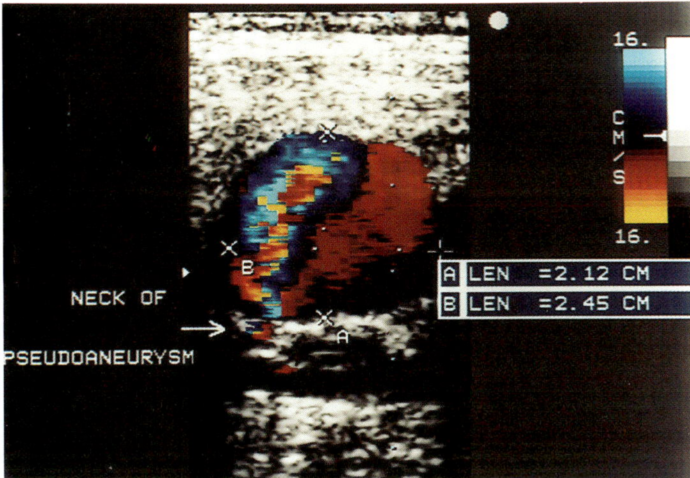

FIGURE 3: *This color duplex ultrasound image of a femoral artery pseudoaneurysm after catheterization reveals the characteristic extraluminal swirling (red and blue) blood flow within the pseudoaneurysm cavity. The cavity measures 2.12 cm vertically by 2.45 cm horizontally.*

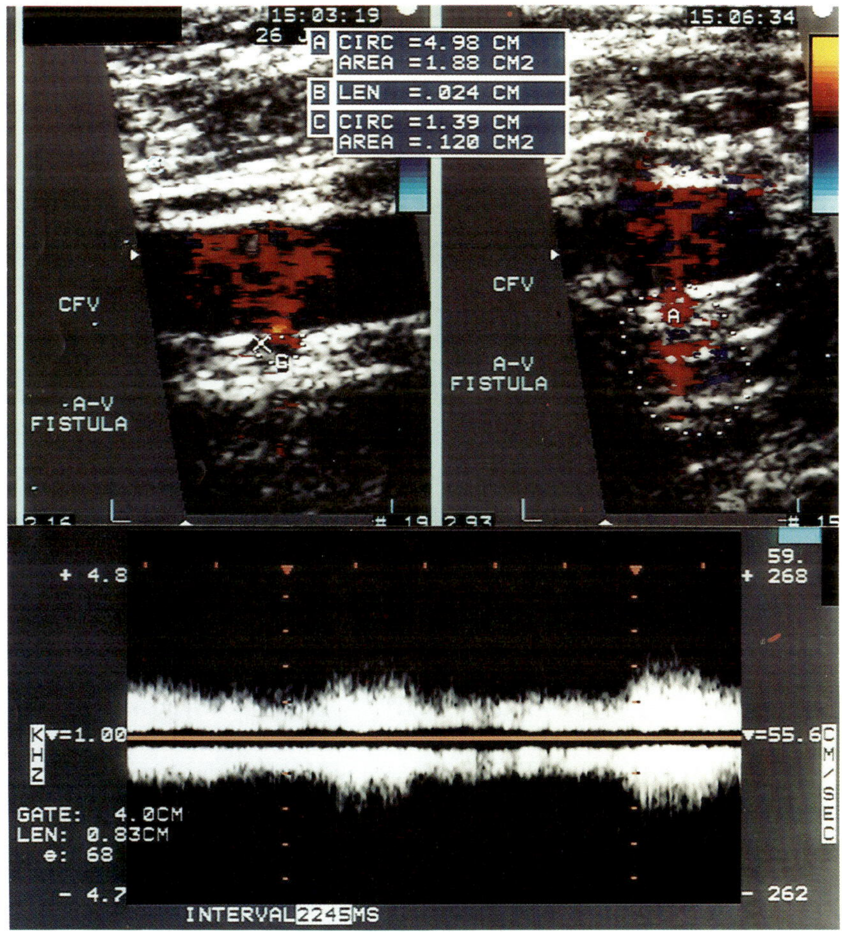

Figure 5: *After catheterization, the color duplex ultrasound images of an arteriovenous fistula reveal the presence of significant arterial to venous flow. In the longitudinal view (upper left panel), a doppler flow jet is seen entering the common femoral vein (CFV). In a transverse view (upper right panel), flow is seen from an arterial branch (A) into the CFV. The Doppler spectrum (lower panel) shows continuous flow throughout the cardiac cycle, which is pathognomonic for arteriovenous fistula.*

V

Future Directions and Conclusions

CHAPTER 10

Intravascular Ultrasound-Imaging in Patients With Coronary Stents

Martin B. Leon, Gary S. Mintz
Gad Keren, Jeffrey J. Popma
Robert F. Bonner

Despite the widespread clinical application of percutaneous transluminal coronary angioplasty (PTCA) several concerns and limitations have impacted on the utilization, safety, and efficacy of this procedure. Balloon-expandable, implantable intracoronary stents have been developed in an effort to improve safety, efficacy, and patency after angioplasty procedures.[1–6] Most stent designs currently in clinical use are poorly visualized with standard angiographic techniques, resulting in poor delineation of the stent and the adjacent vessel wall. Even newer stent designs, composed of more radiopague material such as tantalum,[7] are problematic due to inability to discern lumen features within the radiopaque stent, and inability to "reconstruct" the stent from a three-dimensional perspective. Intravascular ultrasound is a new imaging modality that can help to characterize arterial wall structural changes[8–11] and, due to the highly reflective nature of stent surfaces, can more accurately evaluate alterations in stent geometry. The current study was designed to determine the potential diagnostic applications of intracoronary ultrasound in the acute and long-term follow-up of patients undergoing implantation of metallic coronary stents.

Methods

Patient Population

Eighty-eight patients (mean age 60 ± 13 years) with symptomatic coronary artery disease fulfilling protocol entry criteria for placement of a balloon-

From: Herrmann HC, Hirshfeld JW, eds. *Clinical Use of the Palmaz-Schatz Intracoronary Stent.* Futura Publishing Company, Inc., Mount Kisco, NY, © 1993.

expandable stent participated in the study. There were 72 men and 16 women. The vessel distribution for stent deployment was 22 left anterior descending, 6 circumflex, and 28 right coronary arteries, and 37 saphenous vein grafts. In 72% of patients, stents were implanted at the sites of previous angioplasty restenosis lesions. The mean-minimum lumen diameter for all patients prior to treatment was 0.7 ± 0.5 mm, and the average lesion length was 7.6 ± 4.5 mm. Stents were studied immediately after implantation in 40 patients, 2 to 6 months after implantation (either early symptomatic recurrence or routine angiographic follow-up) in 42 patients, and both acutely and during chronic follow-up evaluation in six other patients.

Intravascular Ultrasound-Imaging Equipment

Ultrasound images were obtained with a mechanical imaging system (InterTherapy, Inc., Costa Mesa, CA) consisting of 1 mm-diameter transducer element, with a center frequency of either 20 or 25 MHz mounted at the distal end of a flexible torque shaft (OD 1.2 mm) within a coronary subselective sheath. Using pulse/echo technique, the ultrasound beam is reflected perpendicular to the catheter-long axis by a mirror positioned at 45°. The received-echo signal was detected, sampled on an 8-bit analog-digital converter, and the scan converted from radial ultrasound-data format into a rectangular format. The image is reviewed on a gray scale video display (Sony) and recorded on a video recorder in real time. The probe is coupled to a motor drive unit, and rotated at 1800 rpm during imaging sequences.

Ultrasound images were obtained after stent placement using either: 1) a 5F-subselective sheath (InterTherapy, Inc.) with a radiopaque tip marker and an inner obturator that was advanced over a standard 0.014-inch or 0.018-inch guidewire; or 2) a 3.9F-monorail-imaging sheath which was interfaced with a motorized catheter-drive module for mechanical pullback of the imaging elements. All arteries were studied in a retrograde fashion from beyond the target lesion into the aorto-ostial junction, either by manual withdrawal of the imaging catheter within the 5F-subselective sheath or using the motorized transducer-pullback device at 0.5 mm per second which permits measurement of axial lengths. At the completion of the imaging study, the imaging catheter and sheath were removed, and repeat angiograms were obtained of the target vessel. There was no evidence of endovascular trauma, thrombus formation, dissection, coronary vasospasm, or reduction in lumen diameter associated with the intracoronary ultrasound-imaging procedures in these patients with coronary stents.

Three-dimensional ultrasound reconstruction of planar images was performed in 10 stents which were implanted in freshly harvested saphenous vein segments, using conventional angioplasty techniques. The 10 in vitro-stent implants represented four different stent designs including: 1) Palmaz-Schatz tubular-slotted balloon-expandable stent (Johnson & Johnson Interventional Systems, Warren, NJ); 2) Wiktor coiled, balloon-expandable tantalum stent

(Medtronic, Inc. Minneapolis, MN); 3) Strecker interlocking-looped, open-mesh balloon-expandable tantalum stent (Boston Scientific Corporation, Boston, MA); and 4) Medinvent woven, self-expanding stainless-steel stent (Schneider, Inc., Minneapolis, MN). Three-dimensional reconstruction was also analyzed in 36 of the aforementioned 88 patients, in whom tubular-slotted balloon-expandable stents were implanted. During in vitro-imaging, an InterTherapy, Inc. intravascular ultrasound system was used. A rotating catheter (at 1800 rpm), consisting of a 25 MHz transducer-tipped, 12-inch-long, rigid probe was withdrawn axially at a pre-determined speed of 0.5 mm per second. In all of the in vivo three-dimensional reconstruction studies, a similar InterTherapy, Inc. intravascular ultrasound system was used, incorporating a 3.9F-monorail-imaging sheath with automated pullback features, at 0.5 mm per second.

Three-dimensional reconstruction of the in vitro and in vivo ultrasound-imaging studies was performed using software developed by Pura, Inc. (Brea, CA) and hardware from ImageComm (Santa Clara, CA). The software-encoded algorithm used binary-thresholding to render the three-dimensional image. The system was set to digitize 7.5 frames per second or 15 cross-sectional image slices/mm of axial stent length. Stent length was measured from the number of seconds (or frames) of video tape in which stent wires appeared; at a motorized transducer-pullback speed of 0.5 mm per second, two seconds of video tape equaled 1 mm of stent length. Gain, offset, threshold, and regions of interest were set to separate the metallic stent from the surrounding vessel wall. The center of rotation was selected to view the stent from the outside to recreate the extracted stent spatial geometry.

Stent Placement Procedures

Tubular-slotted stainless-steel Palmaz-Schatz stents (Johnson & Johnson Interventional Systems, Warren, NJ), were 1.5 cm long (two = 7-mm segments with a central 1-mm-length articulating bridge). The stents were secured on standard or dedicated balloon catheters and were implanted after predilatation, using conventional angioplasty procedures to ensure unencumbered introduction of the more rigid-catheter stent assembly. In the last 50 cases, the stent was placed within either a telescoping subselective sheath (5F or 6F) or a dedicated prepackaged 5F-sheath assembly which was part of a comprehensive stent-delivery system. After stent implantation, subsequent balloon-catheter dilations were frequently necessary to achieve the desired final lumen dimensions.

Ultrasound Image Analysis

The intracoronary ultrasound images were analyzed in a systematic fashion as follows: 1) Reference vessel segments proximal and distal to the stent placement site were studied for lumen dimensions (major diameter, minor diameter, and cross-sectional areas) and vessel wall morphology, including plaque composition; 2) Stents were examined for positioning within the vessel (concentric, eccentric, and shape), circumferential and axial strut expansion, stent-vessel wall contact (circumferential and axial), and lumen dimensions within the stent at various locations (major diameter, minor diameter, and cross-sectional areas). Efforts were made to identify the maximum and minimum stent dimensions within the axial length of the stent as well as all dimensions at the minimum lumen-diameter narrowing, especially for chronic studies. Intimal hyperplasia was calculated from cross-sectional area images and represented the difference between the lumen cross-sectional area and the stent cross-sectional area.

Measurements were made from digitized video recordings using a validated commercial analysis system for diameter and area calculation. When appropriate, comparisons were made between quantitative coronary cineangiographic diameter measurements and corresponding ultrasound images, using branch vessels to identify similar imaging sites.

Quantitative Coronary Angiography

Coronary cineangiograms were analyzed using a validated quantitative angiography system from the Washington Hospital Center Core Angiographic Laboratory. The minimum lumen diameter and percent-diameter stenosis were measured at the stent site and at reference vessel sites. The boundaries of the relevant coronary artery segment were detected automatically from optically magnified, digitized regions of interest of a selected cine-frame. The absolute diameter of stenosis in millimeters is determined by comparison to the known diameter of the guiding catheter.

Results

Angiographic Findings

In all patients, a single stent was successfully deployed per lesion site, and target segments were completely covered by the stent. There were no complications, including acute or subacute thrombotic events, distal embolization, or vasospasm associated with stent placement.

Angiographic results, both acutely and during follow-up examination are detailed in Table 1. Overall, pretreatment minimum lumen diameter increased from 0.72 mm to 2.6 mm, and percent-diameter stenosis was reduced from 76% to 13% after stent implantation. Lumen diameter measurements obtained by angiography immediately after stent placement were consistently lower than final balloon deployment sizes (Fig. 1). The 9% average difference between final balloon diameter and immediate subsequent angiographic lumen diameter represents acute stent recoil. As expected, during follow-up angiography,

Table 1.
Angiographic Results

	Acute QCA		
	IVUS Acute Only (n = 47)	IVUS at Follow-Up: Res (n = 20)	IVUS at Follow-Up: No Res (n = 30)
Pre-minimum lumen diameter (mm)	0.73 ± 0.40	0.64 ± 0.41	0.78 ± 0.42
Pre-lesion length (mm)	7.6 ± 3.0	8.2 ± 3.0	7.8 ± 2.9
Stent size (mm)	3.5 ± 0.4	3.3 ± 0.3	3.3 ± 0.4
Balloon diameter (mm)			
Mean	3.2 ± 0.5	3.2 ± 0.4	3.1 ± 0.5
Minimum	2.7 ± 0.5	2.8 ± 0.4	2.8 ± 0.5
Poststent lumen diameter (mm)			
Mean	2.9 ± 0.5	2.9 ± 0.4	3.0 ± 0.5
Minimum	2.6 ± 0.6	2.5 ± 0.6	2.7 ± 0.5
Reference diameter (mm)	3.0 ± 0.7	3.1 ± 0.5	2.9 ± 0.5

	Follow-Up QCA	
	Res (n = 20)	No Res (n = 30)
Lumen diameter (mm)		
Mean	1.89 ± 0.71	2.21 ± 0.54*
Minimum	0.92 ± 0.72	2.65 ± 0.51*
Reference diameter (mm)	2.82 ± 0.46	2.89 ± 0.48

* $P < 0.001$ vs Res
QCA = quantitative coronary angiography; IVUS = intravascular ultrasound; Res = restensois.

the minimum lumen diameter was considerably lower in the restenosis patients (0.92 mm) compared with the no restenosis patients (2.65 mm, $P < .001$) (Table 1). Interestingly, reference vessel sizes were also slightly reduced in patients during chronic angiographic restudy. Minimum lumen diameter measured by quantitative coronary angiography techniques correlated well with intravascular ultrasound techniques for both acute and chronic studies ($R = 0.69$, $P < .001$).

Ultrasound-Image Analysis

Of the 88 patients studied, ultrasound images were acquired with sufficient resolution to permit careful qualitative and quantitative analysis in all but four patients. These patients were imaged using the larger subselective imaging sheath (5F), and experienced severe ischemia during the course of imaging sequences.

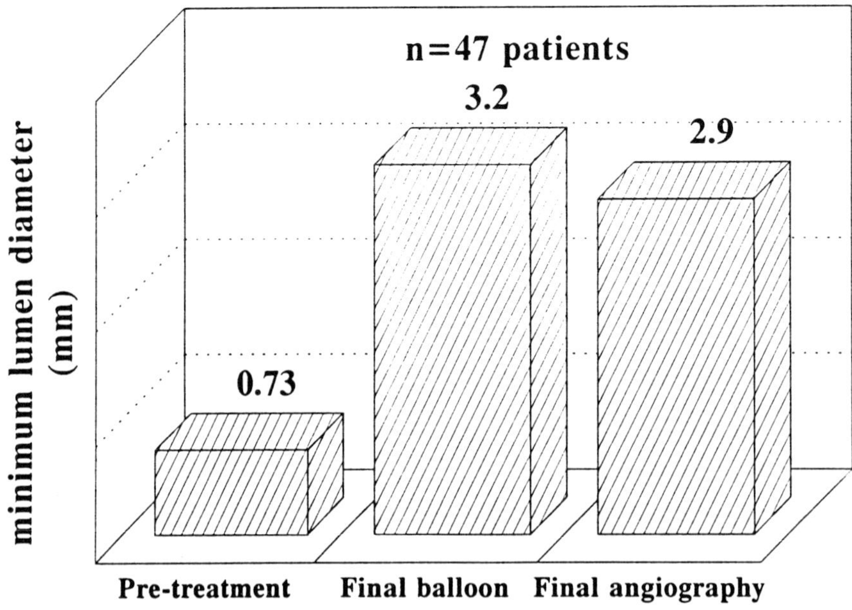

Figure 1: *Quantitative coronary angiographic assessment in 47 patients with stent placement and acute intravascular ultrasound imaging. Bars represent mean values for pretreatment, final expanded balloon, and subsequent final angiography minimum lumen diameters (mm).*

Qualitative Intravascular Ultrasound Observations

In all patients studied, stent struts were detected as bright, highly reflective, hyperechoic "dots" or "dashes", with small subjacent acoustic shadows behind each strut (Fig. 2). Struts could be observed over the complete circumference in most patients, although the interstrut distance (radially) was highly variable. This variability in interstrut distance was likely due to the expanded strut pattern of the stent at the level of the cross-sectional ultrasound plane. However, in some patients, marked coalescence of struts in one region suggests unequal or incomplete expansion of several adjacent strut rows.

The typical morphologic appearance of a stented coronary artery (Fig. 2) consisted of an internal layer of highly reflective stent struts surrounded by an echolucent zone that probably includes compressed and displaced atheroma and media, in part, obscured by acoustic shadowing. A third outer layer that corresponded to the adventitia was seen in all patients. Atheromatous plaque, either below the stent or in reference vessel segments, was detected in all patients, and calcium within atheroma was present in 50% of patients. Of interest, in 74% of patients, atheroma was present in angiographically "normal" proximal vessel segments. Dissection planes or intraluminal-filling de-

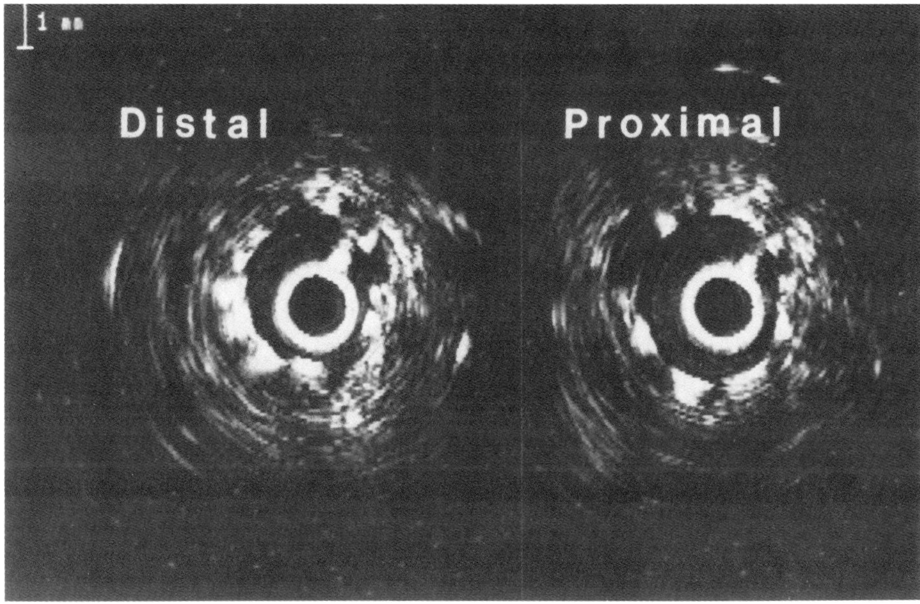

Figure 2: *Distal and proximal stent segments showing stent strut appearance and subjacent vessel wall architecture.*

fects were not detected in stent regions or contiguous vessel segments acutely or during follow-up evaluations of stent implantation.

Quantitative Intravascular Ultrasound (IVUS) Observations

Stent diameters and cross-sectional areas were analyzed demonstrating nonuniform expansion both circumferentially and over the axial length of the stent. An ellipticity score representing the greatest ratio of major to minor diameters was given to individual cross-sectional slices throughout the stent, and indicated significant deformity of stents (ellipticity score greater than 1.5) in approximately 10% of patients acutely (Fig. 3) and during chronic follow-up evaluation (Fig. 4). Axial stent uniformity could be evaluated easily by comparing maximum and minimum stent cross-sectional areas during careful pullback evaluations (Fig. 5). Although stent deformity (ellipticity) implying circumferential nonuniformity was infrequent, significant variations in stent cross-sectional area axially were extremely common. In fact, a nonuniform stent cross-sectional area (ratio of maximum-to-maximum stent cross-sectional area (greater than 1.5) was present in 38% of stents imaged (Fig. 6). The average ratio of maximum-to-minimum stent cross-sectional area for acute studies was 1.43, and for chronic studies it was 1.46.

Importantly, there appear to be subtle but consistent changes in stent

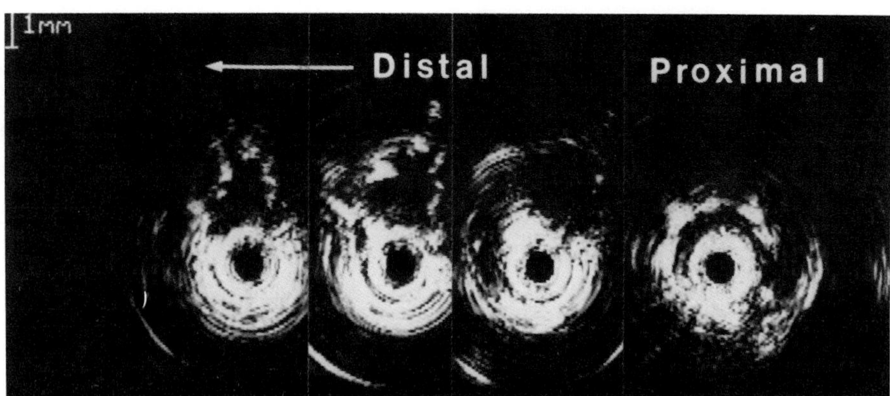

Figure 3: *Pullback through a stent (distal to proximal) showing extreme circumferential nonuniformity with marked compression of superior aspect struts in the distal stent segment after acute implantation.*

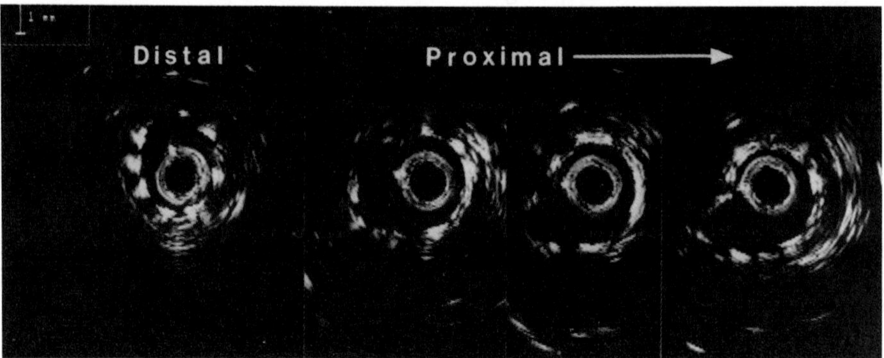

Figure 4: *Nonuniform circumferential appearance of the stent with elliptical deformity of the proximal segment seen during chronic (6-month follow-up) IVUS study.*

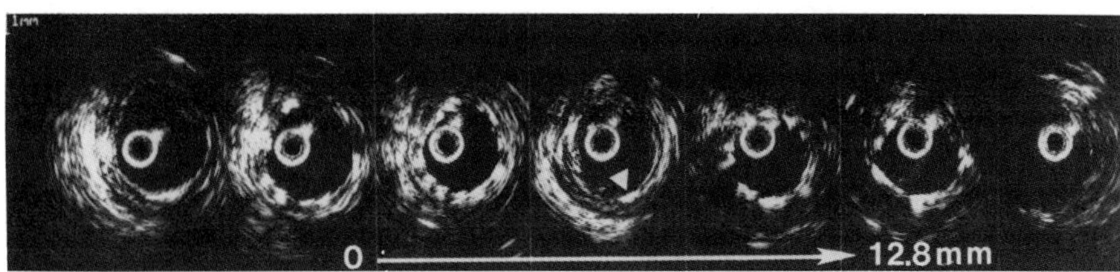

Figure 5: *Selected cross-sectional images from automated pullback demonstrating the ability to assess axial uniformity of stent expansion.*

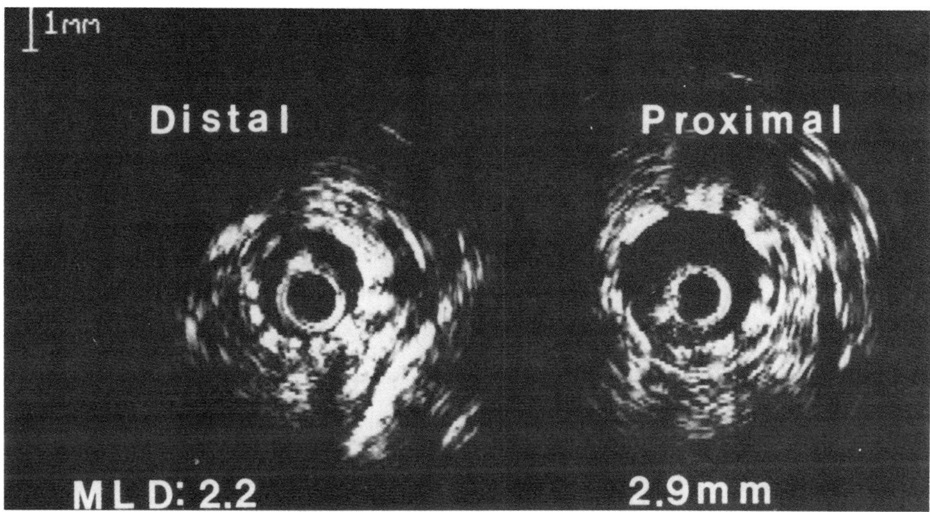

Figure 6: *A fully expanded 3-mm stent showing nonuniform axial expansion with a lesser minimum lumen diameter (interstrut diameter) in the distal versus the proximal stent segment.*

geometry which occur when acute imaging studies are compared with chronic imaging studies. For all stents examined, the minimal stent cross-sectional area decreased from 7.3 ± 2.6 mm^2 to 6.2 ± 2.3 mm^2 in acute versus chronic examinations. This average 15% reduction in minimum stent cross-sectional area was associated with wide interpatient variability, indicating that some patients had excessive late stent narrowing which may have contributed to late lumen loss and restenosis during follow-up studies. Comparing chronic IVUS studies in those patients with versus those without angiographic restenosis (≥ 50%–diameter stenosis), stent dimensions were decreased and intimal hyperplasia was greater in the restenosis subgroup (Fig. 7).

For all chronic intravascular ultrasound images, special consideration was given to detection of tissue growth inside the lumen surface of the stent site representing intimal hyperplasia. The overlying tissue appeared hypoechoic indicating loose highly cellular tissue components in some patients (Fig. 8), but was hyperechoic, suggesting less cellular fibrous components at other stent sites (Fig. 9, top).

Thus, restenosis at stent sites is a complex, multifactorial process involving superficial neointimal formation, resulting in lumen encroachment and geometric deformity of the stent which, in a given patient to a greater or lesser degree, further reduces lumen diameter. Excessive stent compression as the predominant mechanism of restenosis appears uncommon, and may be more frequent in saphenous vein graft lesions (Fig. 10). Depending upon the relative contribution of intimal hyperplasia versus stent compression to restenosis,

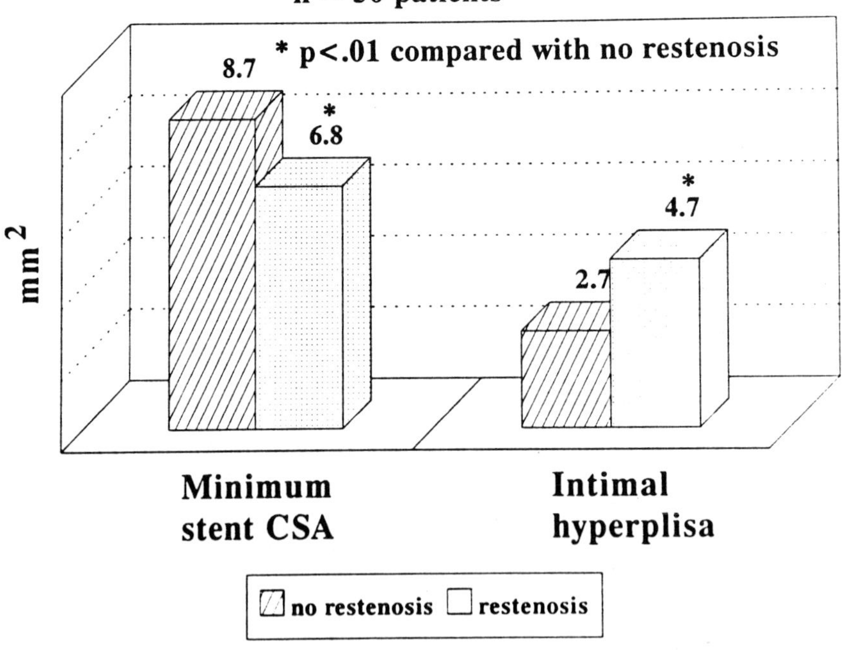

Figure 7: *Comparison of chronic IVUS studies in patients with angiographic restenosis (≥ 50%–diameter stenosis) and those without angiographic restenosis. (Minimum stent cross-sectional area was significantly lower in the restenosis subgroup.) In addition, intimal hyperplasia* **(A)** was significantly greater in the restenosis patients.

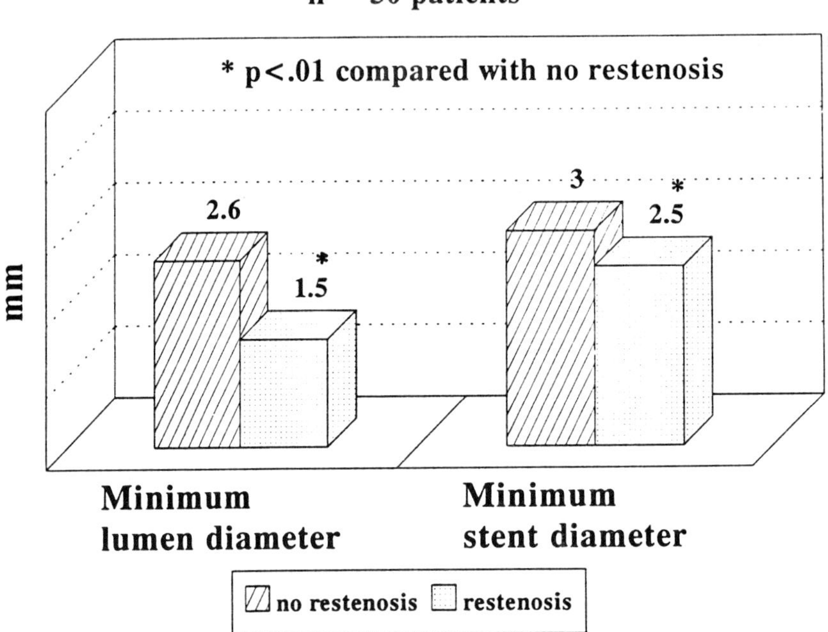

Figure 7B: *Comparison of chronic IVUS studies in patients with angiographic restenosis (≥ 50%–diameter stenosis) and those without angiographic restenosis. (Minimum stent diameter was significantly lower in the restenosis subgroup.)*

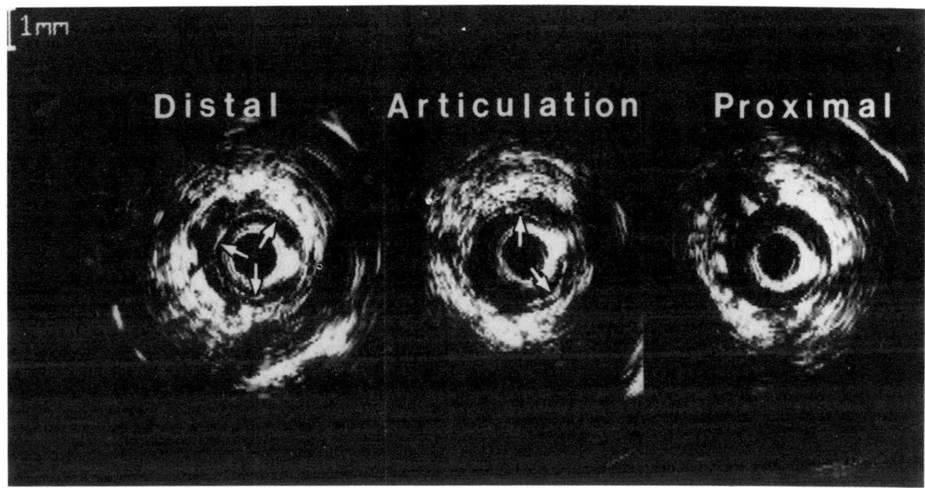

Figure 8: *An example of significant intimal hyperplasia with "soft" hypoechoic tissue overlying the stent struts (distal stent segment).*

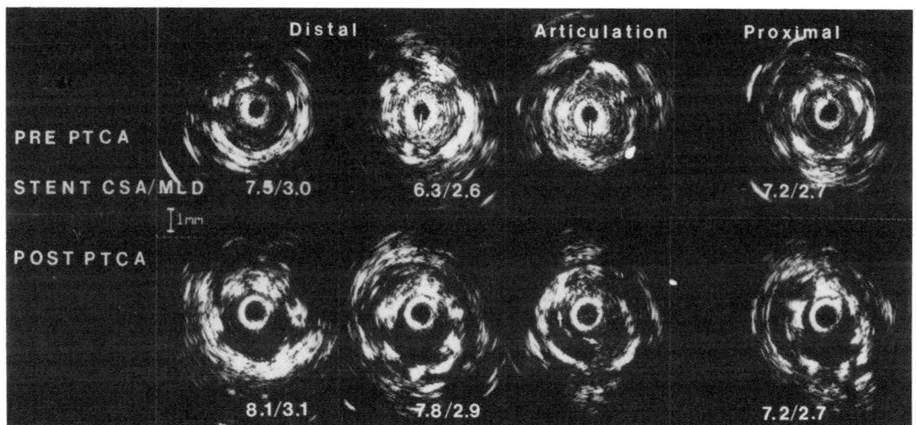

Figure 9: *An example of dense intimal hyperplasia overlying the stent struts in the distal stent segment and at the articulation site. Immediately after balloon angioplasty of this restenotic lesion, there appears to be extrusion of the neointima within the stent and minimal change in actual stent dimensions.*

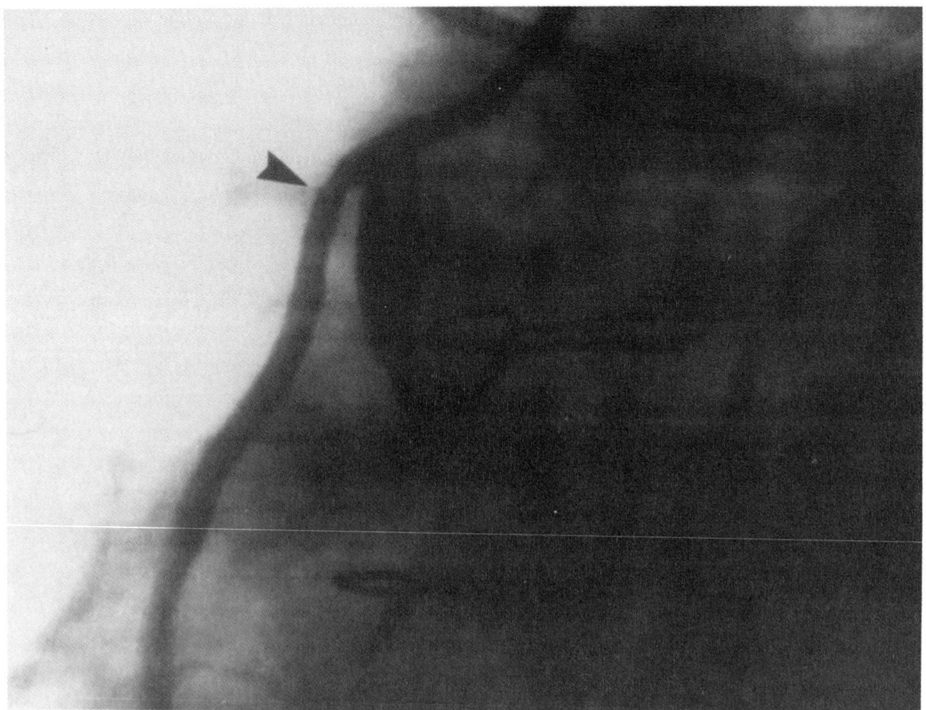

A

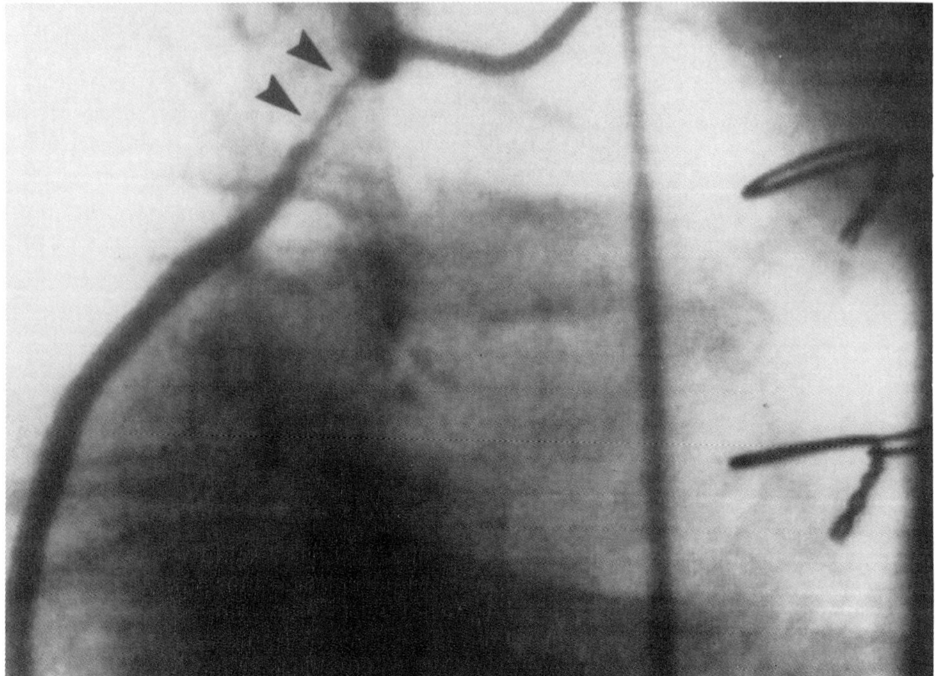

B

Figure 10: *Fully expanded 3-mm stent in the proximal (ostial) location within a saphenous vein graft* **(A)** and subsequent restenosis 2 months later **(B)**.

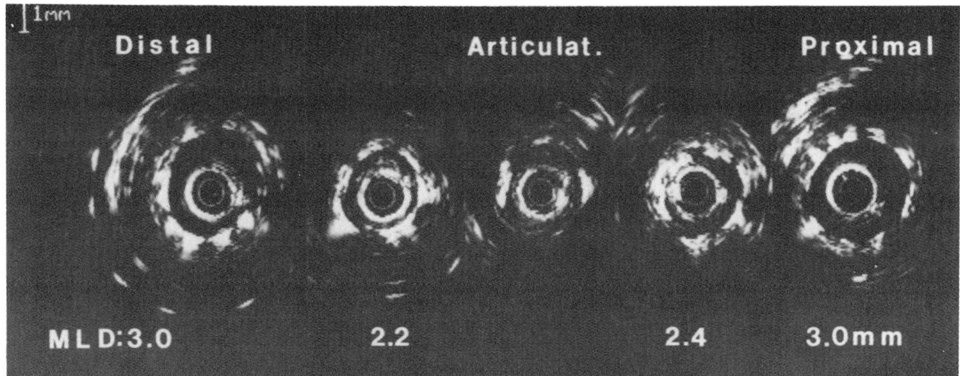

C

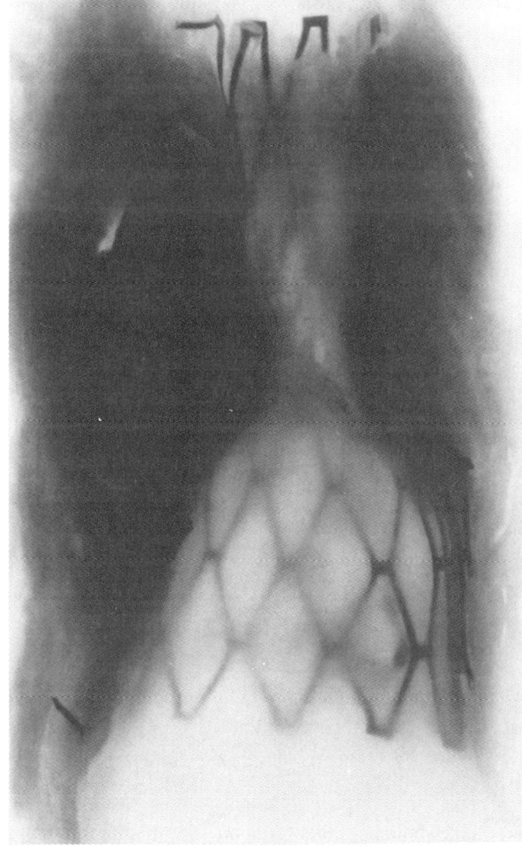

D

Figures 10C,D: *Fully expanded 3-mm stent in the proximal (ostial) location within a saphenous vein graft. Chronic IVUS evaluation of the stent site* **(C)** shows significant reduction in interstrut diameters in addition to intimal hyperplasia contributing to stent restenosis. After repeat surgical revascularization and explanation of the stent, gross pathologic observation shows clear evidence of extrinsic stent compression **(D)**.

PTCA treatment of in-stent narrowing will result in either lumen expansion due to extrusion of neointima through stent struts (Fig. 9) or reexpansion of the narrowed stent itself.

Three-Dimensional Stent Imaging

Three-dimensional reconstruction of cross-sectional intravascular ultrasound image slices of all stents studied in vitro reproduced the aspect ratio and unique spatial geometry of each stent precisely (Fig. 11). In addition, after dissolving tissue, photographs of actual individual stents closely resembled their counterparts obtained by three-dimensional reconstruction of cross-sectional ultrasound image slices.

Three-dimensional reconstruction of intravascular ultrasound images of stents imaged in vivo were similar to those of stents imaged in vitro with a number of exceptions. Cardiac cycle-related vessel motion introduced significant artifacts, and native vessel-vein graft tissue was more echo-dense than freshly excised tissue, making threshold subtraction more difficult. However, in many patients, three-dimensional reconstruction of the ultrasound images did accurately reproduce the stent spatial geometry (Fig. 12).

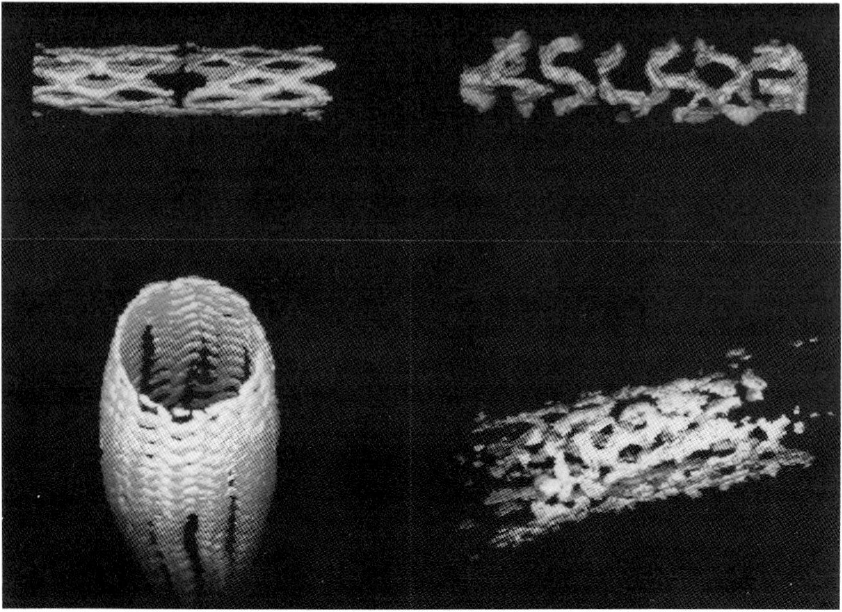

Figure 11: *In vitro intravascular ultrasound three-dimensional reconstruction of four different stent geometries: Palmaz-Schatz stent (top left), Wiktor stent (top right), Medinvent stent (bottom left), and Strecker (bottom right).*

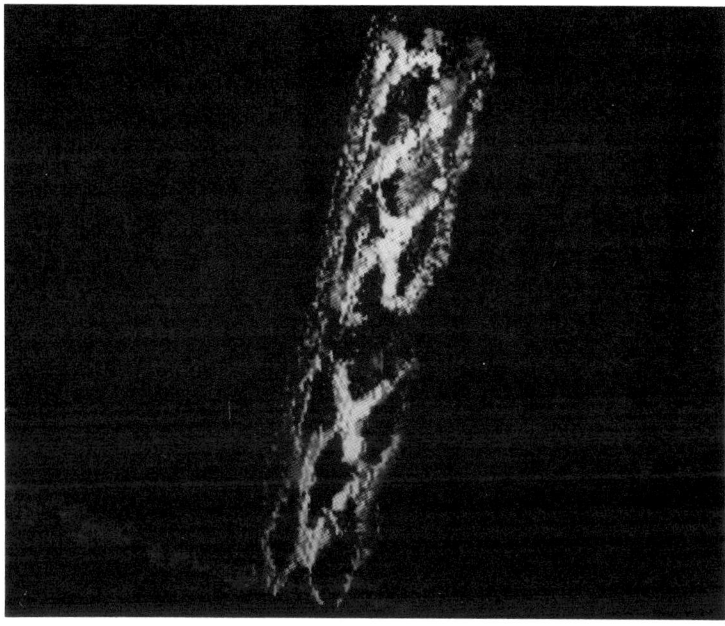

Figure 12: *Three-dimensional in vivo reconstruction of a Palmaz-Schatz stent which was implanted in a mid-right coronary artery. Precise stent geometry and expansion profile are easily discerned in this acute stent implantation study.*

Discussion

Endovascular prosthetic devices have been developed to serve as a scaffold to provide optimal acute patency (opposing recoil of elastic vascular stenosis) and to help reduce the frequency of restenosis. Preliminary reports indicate that stents show promise in reducing complications and improving short and long-term efficacy compared with balloon angioplasty.[12–14]

Previous animal studies have demonstrated an orderly sequence of vessel wall adaptation to the presence of an implanted metallic tubular-slotted stent.[15–19] There is early multicentric endothelialization, which should be completed in several weeks, followed by the formation of a homogeneous neointima and late thinning/atrophy of the media. The ability to examine vessel wall responses after stent implantation in humans has been limited by imaging modalities restricted to contrast angiography. Stainless-steel stents implanted in coronary arteries are effectively radiolucent, and both acute and chronic vessel wall responses have been poorly defined. The use of intravascular ultrasound permits enhanced visual capacity of transmural vessel wall changes after stent implantation. In addition, physical properties and geometry of the stent itself can be clearly determined due to the hyperechoic nature of the stent.

The typical appearance of human coronary stents using intravascular ultrasound imaging consists of an inner region of highly reflective stent struts, which casts small acoustic shadows, a middle hyperechoic region including media and atheroma, and an outer more echogenic adventitia. There is mild circumferential and more significant axial nonuniformity of stent expansion that can be seen both acutely and chronically. These changes are only discerned by ultrasound examination, and are usually sufficiently subtle in magnitude to escape visual angiographic assessment. This implies that stents do not expand in a fully uniform pattern, perhaps due to inhomogeneity of vessel wall compliance, vessel bend points, or anatomical distortion during cardiac motion. Nonuniform strut expansion has also been observed in stents removed from patients.

In addition to nonuniform expansion, stent recoil or compression appears to occur both acutely and after chronic examinations. There is strong evidence that both angiographic and interstrut ultrasound measurements manifest a 10% to 20% reduction in stent diameter immediately upon removal of the final balloon catheter after stent expansion. Over time, as stents adapt to the vessel wall, subsequent lumen compromise is a complex, multifactorial process. In many patients, an echogenic zone of intimal hyperplasia on the luminal surface of the stents can be observed. This certainly accounts for a portion of lumen diameter narrowing noted during follow-up angiography. However, there also appears to be evidence of progressive narrowing of the stent itself with further reduction in measured interstrut diameters by intravascular ultrasound techniques. Importantly, contrast angiography is often unable to differentiate intimal hyperplasia above the stents and intrinsic stent narrowing as a cause of lumen compromise and restenosis. This late "recoil" of the stent may be due to constant stress associated with cardiac motion or vessel tortuosity, mechanical fatigue of the stent strut scaffold, or adjacent luminal hyperplasia resulting in "compression" of the stent from the outer vessel wall.

Interestingly, ultrasound-imaging techniques, combined with mechanical axial catheter withdrawal, and computer software reconstruction permits authentic spatial geometry reconstruction of various stents in three-dimensional pictorial displays. These images should provide unique insights into acute stent deployment factors and chronic adaptive vessel wall responses.

The ultimate role of intravascular ultrasound imaging to assess stent implantation has not been clearly defined. Previous animal studies and peripheral vascular examinations[20,21] suggest that careful ultrasound studies may reveal operator-useful information concerning stent-deployment technique, adverse tissue responses, and mechanisms associated with late lumen narrowing. The pathophysiologic and adaptive responses associated with stent implantation will also undoubtedly effect engineering concepts for future stent designs.

REFERENCES

1. Urban P, Sigwart U, Golf S, Kaufmann U, Sadeghi H, Kappenberger L: Intravascular stenting for stenosis of aortocoronary venous bypass grafts. *J Am Coll Cardiol* 1989; 13:1085–1091.

2. Strauss BH, Serruys PW, Bertrand ME, Puel J, Meier B, Goy JJ, Kappenberger L, Rickards AF, Sigwart U: Quantitative angiographic follow-up of the coronary Wallstent in native vessels and bypass grafts (European experience: March 1986 to March 1990). *Am J Cardiol* 1992; 69:475–481.
3. Schatz RA, Baim DS, Leon M, Ellis SG, Goldberg S, Hirshfeld JW, Cleman MW, Cabin HS, Walker C, Stagg J, Buchbinder M, Teirstein PS, Topol EJ, Savage M, Perez JA, Curry RC, Whitworth H, Sousa E, Tio FO, Almagor Y, Ponder R, Penn IM, Leonard B, Levine SL, Fish RD, Palmaz JC: Clinical experience with the Palmaz-Schatz coronary stent; initial results of a multicenter study. *Circulation* 1991; 83:148–161.
4. Roubin GS, Cannon AD, Agrawal SK, Macander PJ, Dean LS, Baxley WA, Breland J: Intracoronary stenting for acute and threatened closure complicating percutaneous transluminal coronary angioplasty. *Circulation* 1992; 85:916–927.
5. Goy JJ, Sigwart U, Vogt P, Stauffer JC, Kappenberger L: Long-term clinical and angiographic follow-up of patients treated with the self-expanding coronary stent for acute occlusion during balloon angioplasty of the right coronary artery. *J Am Coll Cardiol* 1992; 19:1593–1596.
6. Carrozza JP Jr, Kuntz RE, Levine MJ, Pomerantz RM, Fishman RF, Mansour M, Gibson CM, Senerchia CC, Diver DJ, Safian RD, Baim DS: Angiographic and clinical outcome of intracoronary stenting: immediate and long-term results from a large single-center experience. *J Am Coll Cardiol* 1992; 20:328–337.
7. White CJ, Ramee RR, Banks AK, Mesa JE, Chokshi S, Isner JM: A new balloon-expandable tantalum coil stent: angiographic patency and histologic examination in the atherogenic swine model. *J Am Coll Cardiol* 1992; 19:870–876.
8. Gussenhoven EJ, Essed CE, Lancée CT, Mastik F, Frietman P, van Egmond FC, Reiber J, Bosch H, van Urk H, Roelandt J, Bom N: Arterial wall characteristics determined by intravascular ultrasound imaging: an in vitro study. *J Am Coll Cardiol* 1989; 14:947–952.
9. Nishimura RA, Edwards WD, Warnes CA, Reeder GS, Holmes DR Jr, Tajik AJ, Yock PG: Intravascular ultrasound imaging : in vitro validation and pathologic correlation. *J Am Coll Cardiol* 1990; 16:145–154.
10. Siegel RJ, Fishbein MC, Chae JS, Helfant RH, Hickey A, Forrester JS: Comparative studies of angioscopy and ultrasound for the evaluation of arterial disease. *Echocardiography* 1990; 7:495–502.
11. Potkin BN, Bartorelli AL, Gessert JM, Neville RF, Almagor Y, Roberts WC, Leon MB: Coronary artery imaging with intravascular high frequency ultrasound. *Circulation* 1990; 81:1575.
12. Palmaz JC: Balloon-expandable intravascular stent. *Am J Radiol* 1988; 150:1263.
13. Schatz RA: Introduction to intravascular stents. *Cardiol Clin* 1988; 6:357.
14. Leon MB, Kent KM, Baim DS, Walker CM, Cleman MW, Buchbinder M, Heuser RR, Curry C, Schatz RA, and JJIS Stent Investigators: Comparison of stent implantation in native coronaries and saphenous vein grafts. *J Am Coll Cardiol* 1992; 3: 263A.
15. Schatz RA, Palmaz JC, Tio FO, Garcia F, Garcia O, Reuter SR: Balloon-expandable intracoronary stents in the adult dog. *Circulation* 1987; 76:450–457.
16. Schatz RA: A view of vascular stents. *Circulation* 1989; 79:445.
17. Palmaz JC, Windeler SA, Garcia F, Tio FO, Sibbitt RR, Reuter SR: Atherosclerotic rabbit aortas: expandable intraluminal grafting. *Radiology* 1986; 160:723–726.
18. Robinson KA, Roubin GS, Siegel RJ, Black AJ, Apkarian RP, King SB III: Intra-arterial stenting in the atherosclerotic rabbit. *Circulation* 1988; 78:646–653.
19. Bartorelli AL, Neville RF, Almagor Y, Perlman MW, Leon MB: Intravascular catheter-based ultrasound: in vivo imaging of artery wall and stents. *Circulation* 1989; 80:II-580.
20. Chokshi SK, Hogan J, Dasai V, Daod M, Cross F, Parsonnet V, Isner JM: Intravascular ultrasound assessment of implanted endovascular stents. *J Am Coll Cardiol* 1990; 15:29A.
21. Isner JM, Rosenfeld K, Losordo D, Kelly S, Palefski P, Langevin RE, Razvi SK, Pastore JO, Kosowsky BD: Percutaneous intravascular ultrasound as adjunct to catheter-based interventions: preliminary experience in patients with peripheral vascular disease. *Radiology* 1990; 175:61–70.

CHAPTER 11

Clinical Use of the Palmaz-Schatz Stent in Perspective: Suggested Indications

Stephen G. Ellis

The proper role of any new therapy must be judged on the basis of its risk to benefit ratio when compared to that of other potential treatments. Intracoronary stenting holds considerable promise for treatment of poor initial angioplasty (PTCA) results and to limit the likelihood of restenosis.[1–3] With currently available data, and acknowledging the limitations of its nonrandomized origin, one can now make a reasonable attempt to assess the risk to benefit ratio of stenting relative to PTCA for both elective and nonelective therapy. However, due to the explosion of new technologies competitive with PTCA (directional and rotational atherectomy, excimer laser, etc.), assessing the likely overall role of stenting is somewhat speculative.

Potential Indication: Treatment of Suboptimal Percutaneous Transluminal Coronary Angioplasty Result

Leaving behind an angiographically apparent dissection of 25% to 49% stenosis after PTCA clearly heightens the risk of major in-hospital ischemic complications (death, urgent bypass surgery, or myocardial infarction) by a factor of two- to fivefold.[4–6] Dissections greater than 10 to 15 mm, transient total occlusion, extraluminal contrast staining, and more severe residual stenosis heighten that risk.[5] Prolonged balloon inflation, often with a perfusion balloon, appears to reduce the risk of these complications consequent to major dissection by about one-third, but adverse outcomes may still occur in as many as half of high-risk patients.[7,8]

Interest in electively placing a stent to improve luminal dimensions and blood flow, and to "tack up" a tear or dissection has thus naturally arisen. It

From: Herrmann HC, Hirshfeld JW, eds. *Clinical Use of the Palmaz-Schatz Intracoronary Stent.* Futura Publishing Company, Inc., Mount Kisco, NY, © 1993.

is uncertain, however, whether or not it is "worth" taking the risk of stenting (subacute thrombosis, hemorrhage, and the added cost of the procedure) for all or some of these patients. Of the first 738 patients with attempted Palmaz-Schatz native vessel stent placement, 315 lesions were stented for a "suboptimal result," and this stent is under FDA consideration for approval for this indication.

What do we know about this group of patients and lesions, and how they might have fared without stenting? One hundred-fourteen lesions had greater than or equal to a 50% stenosis after PTCA but no obvious dissection, 75 lesions had a dissection with a less than a 50% residual stenosis, and 75 lesions had both a dissection and a significant residual stenosis. Incomplete information is available for the remaining 51 lesions. The 30-day outcome for these patients and lesions is quite favorable as shown in Table 1. However, since physicians deliberately undersize dilatation balloons prior to stent delivery, many patients in the "residual stenosis only" group may simply have been underdilated. Furthermore, the lengths of the dissections have not been described, and there is no way to assess the risk of vessel closure without stenting in this group.

How can we attempt to resolve this important issue? Outcome from a randomized trial would be helpful, but is not likely to be forthcoming. One can attempt to extrapolate from data with other stents, although the delivery ease and luminal result after implantation of different stents are not equal.[9] In the absence of a randomized trial, Lincoff and colleagues have attempted to clarify this issue by performing a case-control study.[10] Patients with threatened closure or true closure treated with a Gianturco-Roubin stent were matched on the basis of prognostic criteria to patients with similar characteristics treated just before the availability of that stent at the same institutions. In that analysis of 122-patient outcomes, patients with true closure treated early (≥ 45 minutes) with stents could be shown to benefit, but patients treated late or with threatened closure only (TIMI 3 flow) did not appear to be helped. More-

Table 1.
Treatment of "Suboptimal PTCA Result"*

n = 315 lesions	
Successful implant	97.5%
No dissection, poststent < 50% residual stenosis	80.1%
Death ≤ 30 days	0.6%
Urgent CABG	
Dissection group	5.3%
No dissection group	1.8%
Nonfatal MI	2.6%
Stent thrombosis	
Dissection group	4.7%
No dissection group	7.9%

* Dissection and/or post-PTCA stenosis > 50%
Source: Johnson and Johnson Interventional Systems, Inc. (JJIS) Database, 1992
PTCA = percutaneous transluminal coronary angioplasty; CABG = coronary artery bypass grafts.

Table 2.
Suggested Indications* for Palmaz-Schatz Stent Placement for "Suboptimal Result"

Definite
> 50% diameter stensosis despite ≥ 10 m inflation with appropriately sized balloon, artery ≥ 3.0 mm and artery or patient not well-suited for directional atherectomy

Probable
Threatened closure with certain high-risk characteristics:
Dissection ≥ 10–15 mm but residual stenosis < 50%, artery ≥ 3.0 mm
Persistent ≥ 50% stenosis, artery ≥ 3.0 mm

Possible
Lower risk threatened closure or small artery
Dissection < 10–15 mm, artery ≥ 3.0 mm
Persistent 40–49% stenosis, artery ≥ 3.0 mm
Dissection ≥ 10–15 mm, artery 2.5–2.9 mm
Persistent > 50% stenosis, artery 2.5–2.9 mm
High risk of restenosis in a major artery
Persistent > 30% residual stenosis

Definitely Not
Recent major organ system bleeding (except with life-threatening true closure)
Artery < 2.5 mm (except as a bridge to surgery)

* Including use as a bridge to surgery if stent closure would be imminently life-threatening, or if risk of bleeding is high.

over, those stented for threatened closure received more blood product transfusions and were hospitalized longer than their nonstented counterparts.

For patients with a suboptimal result due to a dissection and a moderate residual stenosis after PTCA (25% to 49%), the high risk of restenosis of 40% to 50%[11] must be considered, in addition to the risks of in-hospital ischemic complications. Devices other than balloons and stents may be used in this setting. Directional atherectomy has been reported in small series to have an 85% to 90% likelihood of procedural success, but the risk of perforation may be as high as 3%.[12,13] Furthermore, this strategy often requires a guide-catheter exchange with possible loss of guidewire position and, thus, seems to have limited applicability. Mid-range (50 to 60°C) thermal balloons[14] and temporary stents[15] are in the early clinical testing phase and may be useful in this setting.

In summary, the indications for Palmaz-Schatz stent implantation for a suboptimal PTCA result remain unclear. True abrupt closure has very serious consequences and should be prevented, but selection of patients with threatened closure at greatest risk of closure or late restenosis, and of patients for whom stenting will be beneficial remains problematic. Suggested indications for the use of a Palmaz-Schatz stent in this setting are provided in Table 2.

Potential Indication: Prevention of Restenosis in De Novo Lesions

The cost of treating patients in the United States alone for restenosis was estimated to be 3.8 billion dollars in 1990,[16] and will only increase as more angioplasties are performed and as the medical cost of treatment likewise increases. No medical treatment to prevent restenosis has convincingly been shown to be beneficial, although pretreatment for several days to weeks with fish oil supplements or HMG CoA-reductase inhibitors appears to show promise.[17,18]

Risk factors for restenosis have been analyzed,[16,18] and this analysis has allowed the development of nomograms which identify patients at highest risk; these patients would be most likely to gain from an intervention that successfully reduces restenosis. In meta-analyses of clinically-associated variables, variant angina (odds ratio = 2.7), diabetes (odds ratio = 2.1), continued smoking (odds ratio = 2.0), new onset angina (odds ratio = 1.5), and possibly male gender (odds ratio = 1.4) seem to be the most important ones.[16] In similar meta-analyses of angiographic variables, proximal vessel location (odds ratio = 1.4), left anterior descending location (odds ratio = 1.4), and saphenous vein graft location (odds ratio = 1.4) appear to increase the risk of restenosis.[16] The large M-HEART study[11] found that lesion length, graft or left anterior descending artery (LAD) location, pre-PTCA percent stenosis, eccentricity, and native artery diameter each independently affected outcome. Procedural variables such as balloon sizing and final angiographic result were also important,[11] but could not be predicted beforehand.

In the absence of a randomized trial result to draw on, the Johnson and Johnson Interventional Systems, Inc. (JJIS) Stent Registry provides the best information about long-term angiographic follow-up and restenosis following placement of the Palmaz-Schatz stent; results with other stents are likely to be different.[9,19] The registry results are summarized in Tables 3 to 5. Delivery success was high (> 95%) and early complications rather low when stents were implanted electively (Table 3). Early risk was particularly low for saphenous vein graft implants, despite their mean age of 8 years. The incidence of

Table 3.
Delivery Success and 30-Day Outcome

	Native Vessels (n = 738 pts.)	*Vein Grafts (n = 276 pts.)*
Successful implant	95.9%	97.5%
Death	0.5%	0.7%
Urgent CABG	2.6%	0.7%
Elective CABG	0.1%	0.7%
Nonfatal MI	2.2%	2.5%
Stroke	0.1%	0.4%
Stent thrombosis	6.0%	0.7%
Stent embolization—coronary	0.1%	0.0%
peripheral	1.7%	0.0%
Hemorrhage requiring transfusion or repair	11.1%	NR

Source: JJIS Database
CABG = coronary artery bypass grafts; MI = myocardial infarction.

Table 4.
Rates of Restenosis in Native Vessels

n = 484 patients (90% angiographic follow-up)		
Overall	29.8%	
Prior restenosis		
Yes	33.5%	*P* = 0.02
No	21.1%	
Multiple stents		
Yes	45.9%	*P* < 0.001
No	26.3%	
Reference diameter		
< 3.0 mm	37.0%	*P* = 0.006
≥ 3.0 mm	27.2%	
Poststent diameter		
< 3.0 mm	38.0%	*P* < 0.001
≥ 3.0 mm	26.8%	
Ideal (de novo, ≥ 3.0 mm diameter, short)		
Yes	11.0%	*P* < 0.001
No	34.1%	

Source: JJIS Database, 1992

restenosis in both native arteries and vein grafts within 6 months was lowest for short, de novo lesions in arteries greater than or equal to 3.0 mm in diameter, particularly if an excellent angiographic result was obtained after stenting (Tables 4, 5). These results appear to be sustained when angiographic follow-up is continued to 12 months.[20]

More detailed information is available for the first 200 patients who received the Palmaz-Schatz stent in native arteries[3] and also the first 86 patients who received stents for saphenous vein stenoses.[21] The placement of multiple overlapping stents for long lesions in an attempt to prevent restenosis cannot be condoned, on the basis of an observed 46% to 64% restenosis rate.[3] However, data with single stents are more promising. These data, originating from the core angiographic laboratory at Thomas Jefferson University, found that the "average" de novo native LAD stenosis stented was 7 mm in length, was eccentric 45% of the time, was located in a 3.2-mm artery and initially had a 71%–diameter narrowing. Based upon the M-HEART data, the probability of restenosis in this lesion would be 39%, yet only 14% (95% confidence interval = 8% to 20%) developed restenosis (Table 6). Similar comparison for de novo native right or circumflex coronary arteries (mean lesion length = 7 mm, eccentric in 41%, reference diameter = 3.3, 79% stenosis) found an expected restenosis rate of about 28%, and an actual rate of 13% (95% confidence interval 10–17%). For de novo vein graft lesions (mean lesion length = 5 mm, eccentric in 50%, reference diameter 3.7 mm, 83% stenosis) the expected restenosis rate

Table 5.
Rates of Restenosis in Vein Grafts

n = 149 patients		
Overall	28.9%	
Prior restenosis		
Yes	40.9%	$P < 0.001$
No	17.9%	
Multiple stents		
Yes	33.3%	P = NS
No	27.9%	
Reference diameter		
< 3.0 mm	57.9%	$P < 0.001$
≥ 3.0 mm	24.2%	
Ideal (de novo, ≥ 3.0 mm diameter, short)		
Yes	16.9%	$P < 0.001$
No	36.7%	

Source: JJIS Database, 1992

was 68% while that observed was only 18% (95% confidence interval 14% to 22%) (Table 6).

This analysis is limited in that it may not take into account other factors biasing the operator to attempt stent implantation (all of these patients could have simply been treated with PTCA). Of recognized risk factors not included in the M-HEART-based analysis, the higher incidence of diabetes in the stented population compared with that in data used for the meta-analysis (19% versus 8%) might possibly balance the impact of a lesser incidence of continued smoking (13% versus 52%), but it must be acknowledged that the "science" of this

Table 6.
Restenosis *Observed* in Stented Patients (n = 633) vs. *Expected* in Routine PTCA*

	Observed (%)	*Expected (%)*
De novo LAD/1 stent	14 (8–20)	*39 (27–51)*
De novo LCX or RCA/1 stent	13 (10–17)	*28 (16–40)*
De novo vein graft/1 stent	18 (14–22)	*68 (60–76)*
Restenotic LAD/1 stent	31 (26–36)	*37 (24–50)*
Restenotic LCX or RCA/1 stent	31 (28–34)	*22 (11–33)*
Restenotic vein graft/1 stent	41 (35–47)	*50 (47–63)*

* Observed with 95% confidence intervals; expected with 95% confidence intervals per M-HEART data[11] matched for diameter, length, pre-PTCA %-stenosis and eccentricity (native vessels) or literature search (vein grafts).
PTCA = percutaneous transluminal coronary angioplasty; LAD = left anterior descending artery; LCX = left cirumflex; RCA = right coronary artery.

method of comparison is crude. The Registry data includes the early experience, when it was not widely recognized that a nearly perfect poststent result was required to optimize protection from restenosis. For example, the risk of restenosis with a single stent and final percent stenosis less than or equal to 0% was a remarkably low 6%, while if such an angiographic result was not achieved, the restenosis rate was 33%.[3] Thus, the data used in the above comparison may represent a worst-case scenario for the Palmaz-Schatz stent. We expect a much more accurate appraisal of benefit from the ongoing randomized STRESS trial comparing single stent implantation to PTCA in de novo lesions in arteries greater than or equal to 3.0 mm in diameter.

The risk and cost of stenting also must be considered in a comparison of stenting and routine PTCA. The risk of bleeding and local vascular complications after stenting is increased, compared with PTCA. Subacute thrombosis occurs in 1% to 6% of patients,[22] most commonly 3 days to 3 weeks after implantation, and often results in total occlusion and infarction just after the patient has left the hospital. This problem is rare after routine PTCA, and must be considered the major limitation of stenting at present. Stenting is generally avoided in patients at heightened risk of bleeding (those with recently active gastritis or peptic ulcer disease, for example) or thrombosis (true aspirin allergy). Bleeding, local groin complications, and the time to achieve stable anticoagulation times with warfarin all add to the cost of the procedure. Data from the early stent experience suggested that stenting might result in hospital charges exceeding those of PTCA by almost $8000![23] Even assuming that further experience could reduce this excess by 50%, the restenosis rate would have to be reduced from about 40% to 20% to 25% to financially "break even".[16] One approach to reducing the cost of stenting is to use a brachial approach with the patient already anticoagulated.[24] If such an approach can be proven safe in larger numbers of patients (a study is currently underway), then cost might become less of an impediment to the strategy of elective stent placement.

Other strategies to reduce restenosis that may have lower bleeding and cost complications include atherectomy and the excimer laser. The excimer laser, thus far, has been associated with rates of restenosis even higher than seen with PTCA.[25] Rotational, directional, and extraction atherectomy, although not quite as well studied in this regard, are similarly not promising.[26–28] The effect of directional atherectomy on restenosis is being studied in the CAVEAT trial. Hence, among the currently assessed new mechanical technologies, only stenting holds considerable promise to decrease the incidence of the "Achilles heel" of angioplasty.

In my opinion, placement of a single Palmaz-Schatz stent for the indication to prevent restenosis in a de novo lesion appears to be very reasonable for LAD and saphenous vein graft stenoses, based upon the apparent remarkable reduction in restenosis rates compared to those reported for PTCA alone. Right and left circumflex artery stenoses have generally lower restenosis rates with PTCA, and less apparent benefit with stenting (see above); clear benefit from a randomized comparison should be demonstrated before stenting can be advo-

Table 7.
Suggested Indications for Stenting of De Novo Lesions to Prevent Restenosis

Definite
None
Probable
Focal LAD or saphenous vein graft lesions in arteries ≥ 3.0 mm
Possible
Focal LCX or RCA lesions in arteries ≥ 3.0 mm
Focal LAD or saphenous vein graft lesions in arteries 2.6–2.9 mm
Definitely Not
Lesions requiring placement of multiple overlapping stents
Lesions in arteries ≤ 2.5 mm
Lesions for which closure would be imminently life-threatening (e.g., unprotected left main stenosis)
Patients at heightened risk of bleeding

LAD = left anterior descending artery; LCX = left cirumflex; RCA = right coronary artery.

cated in these arteries. Suggested indications for stenting de novo lesions to prevent restenosis are shown in Table 7.

Potential Indication: Prevention of Restenosis in Previously Restenotic Lesions

Many of the arguments described in the previous section apply to an analysis of stenting to prevent re-restenosis, but unfortunately the data are even more wanting. Nomograms predictive of outcome after PTCA are not as well developed. A single recurrence does not appear to increase the risk by more than 5% to 10%, unless it occurs within the first 4 to 5 months after PTCA.[16,29] However, a second or further restenosis increases the likelihood of a subsequent restenosis considerably, probably to about 50%.[30] Interestingly, while a single restenosis dramatically increases the risk of restenosis after stenting to about 35%,[3] multiple restenoses seem to have a much lesser incremental effect.[31] For restenotic lesions after conventional PTCA, the Registry data suggest a restenosis rate for a single stent of 25% to 31% in the LAD (but 50% for the proximal LAD), of 29% to 31% for the left circumflex (LCX) or right coronary artery (RCA), and of 41% for saphenous vein grafts,[3,21] but the confidence intervals for these figures are wide (Table 6).

Presently, the author would favor withholding stent placement for this indication unless: 1) initial PTCA yielded a poor result that was not amenable to other therapies that might improve the result without the risks of stent placement (directional or rotational atherectomy); or 2) the lesion had recurred more than once; or 3) randomized trials suggest a benefit for a wider range of indications. These suggestions are summarized in Table 8.

Table 8.
Suggested Indications for Elective for Stenting of Restenotic Lesions to Prevent Restenosis

Definite
  None
Probable
  Poor initial PTCA result, not amenable to treatment with other new devices with lesser risk of bleeding than stents, artery ≥ 3.0 mm
  Recurrrent restenosis in a artery of major importance, artery ≥ 3.0 mm
Possible
  Any restenosis in artery ≥ 3.0 mm
  Poor initial PTCA result, not amenable to treatment with other new devices with lesser risk of bleeding than stents, artery 2.6–2.9 mm
Definitely Not
  Lesions that would require placement of multiple overlappping stents
  Lesions in arteries ≤ 2.5 mm
  Lesions for which closure would be imminently life-threatening (e.g., unprotected left main stenosis
  Patients at heightened risk of bleeding

PTCA = percutaneous transluminal coronary angioplasty.

Conclusions

In suitably-selected patients, delivery success is excellent for the Palmaz-Schatz coronary stent. Its use appears very promising as a method of improving suboptimal PTCA results, and to decrease the likelihood of restenosis in selected patients. This impression is, however, based solely upon analysis of registry-based data, and cannot be considered conclusive until appropriate controlled studies are performed. Use of the Palmaz-Schatz stent in emergent situations, e.g., to rescue a failed PTCA complicated by acute vessel closure, was not specifically studied in the registry. Data from a small group of patients receiving stents for this indication and suggested guidelines for its use are presented in Chapter 6.

REFERENCES

1. Sigwart U, Urgan P, Golf S, Kaufmann U, Imbert C, Fischer A, Kappenberger L: Emergency stenting for acute occlusion after coronary balloon angioplasty. *Circulation* 1988; 78:1121–1127.
2. Roubin GS, Cannon AD, Agrawal SK, Macander PJ, Dean LS, Baxley WA, Breland J: Intracoronary stenting for acute and threatened closure complicating percutaneous transluminal coronary angioplasty. *Circulation* 1992; 85:916–927.
3. Ellis SG, Savage M, Fischman D, Baim DS, Leon M, Goldberg S, Hirshfeld JW, Cleman MW, Teirstein PS, Walker C, Bailey S, Buchbinder M, Topol EJ, Schatz RA: Restenosis after placement of Palmaz-Schatz stents in native coronary arteries: initial results of a multicenter experience. *Circulation* 1992; 86:1836–1844.

4. Ellis SG, Roubin GS, King SB, Douglas JS Jr, Weintraub WS, Thomas RG, Cox WR: Angiographic and clinical predictors of acute closure after native vessel coronary angioplasty. *Circulation* 1988; 77:372–379.
5. Black AJR, Namay DL, Niederman AL, Lembo NJ, Roubin GS, Douglas JR, King SB: Tear or dissection after coronary angioplasty: morphologic correlates of an ischemic complication. *Circulation* 1989; 79:1035–1042.
6. Huber MS, Mooney JF, Madison J, Mooney MR: Use of a morphologic classification to predict clinical outcome after dissection from coronary angioplasty. *Am J Cardiol* 1991; 68:467–471.
7. Leitschuh ML, Mills RM, Jacobs AK, Ruocco NA, LaRosa D, Faxon DP: Outcome after major dissection during coronary angioplasty using the perfusion balloon catheter. *Am J Cardiol* 1991; 67:1056–1060.
8. Lincoff AM, Popma JJ, Ellis SG, Hacker JA, Topol EJ: Abrupt vessel closure complicating coronary angioplasty: clinical angiographic and therapeutic profile. *J Am Coll Cardiol* 1992; 19:926–935.
9. Ellis SG, Verlee P, Muller DW: Comparison of outcome after slotted tube vs. coil stainless steel coronary stent implantation to prevent restenosis. *Circulation* (submitted for publication).
10. Lincoff AM, Topol EJ, Chapekis AT, George BS, Candela RJ, Muller DWM, Zimmerman CA, Ellis SG: Intracoronary stenting compared with conventional therapy for abrupt vessel closure complicating coronary angioplasty: a matched case-control study. *J Am Coll Cardiol* 1993; 21:866–875.
11. Hirshfeld JW, Schwartz JS, Jugo R, MacDonald RG, Goldberg S, Savage MP, Bass TA, Vetrovec G, Cowley M, Taussig AS, Whitworth HG, Margolis JR, Hill JA, Pepine CJ and M-HEART Investigators: Restenosis after coronary angioplasty: a multivariate statistical model to relate lesion and procedure variables to restenosis. *J Am Coll Cardiol* 1991; 18:647–656.
12. Whitlow PL, Robertson GC, Rowe MH, Douglas JS, Cowley MJ, Kereiakes CJ, Smucker ML, Hartzler GO, Hinohara T: Directional coronary atherectomy for failed percutaneous transluminal coronary angioplasty. *Circulation* 1990; 82:III-1. Abstract.
13. Vetter JW, Simpson JB, Robertson GC, Selmon MR, Rowe MH, Bartzokis TC, Braden LJ, Hinohara T: Rescue directional coronary atherectomy for failed balloon angioplasty. *J Am Coll Cardiol* 1991; 17:384A. Abstract.
14. Fram DB, Aretz TA, Fisher JP, Milkan JS, Reisner A, Mitchel JF, Gillam LD, McKay RG: In vivo radiofrequency balloon angioplasty of porcine coronary arteries: histologic effects and safety. *J Am Coll Cardiol* 1992; 19:217A. Abstract.
15. Whitlow P, Gaspard P, Kent K, Baim D, Chapman J, Heuser R, Knopf W: Improvement of coronary dissection with a removable flow support catheter: acute results. *J Am Coll Cardiol* 1992; 19:217A. Abstract.
16. Califf RM, Ohman EM, Frid DJ, Fortin DF, Mark DB, Hlatky MA, Herndon JE, Bengtson JR: Restenosis: the clinical issues. In: Topol EJ, ed. *Textbook of Interventional Cardiology*. Philadelphia: W.B. Saunders Co; 1990:363–394.
17. Dehmer GJ, Popma JJ, van den Berg EK, Eichhorn EJ, Prewitt JB, Campbell WB, Jennings L, Willerson JT, Schmitz JM: Reduction in the rate of early restenosis after coronary angioplasty by a diet supplemented with n-3 fatty acids. *N Engl J Med* 1988; 319:733–740.
18. Popma JJ, Califf RM, Topol EJ: Clinical trials of restenosis after coronary angioplasty. *Circulation* 1991; 84:1426–1436.
19. Serruys PW, Strauss BH, Beatt IV, Bertrand ME, Puel J, Rickards AF, Meier B, Goy JJ, Vogt P, Kappenberger L, Sigwart U: Angiographic follow-up after placement of a self-expanding coronary artery stent. *N Engl J Med* 1991; 324:13–17.
20. Savage M, Fischman D, Ellis S, Leon M, Cleman M, Teirstein P, Walker C, Hirshfeld J, Schatz R, Goldberg S: Does late progression of restenosis occur beyond six months following coronary artery stenting? *Circulation* 1990; 82:III-540.

21. Leon MB, Kent KM, Baim DS, Walker CM, Cleman MW, Buchbinder M, Heuser RR, Curry C, Schatz RA, and JJIS Stent Investigators: Comparison of stent implantation in native coronaries and saphenous vein grafts. *J Am Coll Cardiol* 1992; 19: 263A.
22. Schatz RA, Baim DS, Leon M, Ellis SG, Goldberg S, Hirshfeld JW, Cleman MW, Cabin HS, Walker C, Stagg J, Buchbinder M, Tierstein PS, Topol EJ, Savage M, Perez JA, Curry RC, Whitworth H, Sousa JE, Tio FO, Almagor Y, Ponder LR, Penn IM, Leonard B, Levine SL, Fish D, Palmaz JC: Clinical experience with the Palmaz-Schatz coronary stent: initial results of a multicentsr study. *Circulation* 1991; 83: 148–161.
23. Dick RJ, Popma JJ, Muller DWM, Burek KA, Topol EJ: In-hospital costs associated with new percutaneous coronary devices. *Am J Cardiol* 1991; 68:879–885.
24. Rosenschein U, Ellis SG: Preprocedure warfarinization and brachial approach for elective coronary stent placement: a possible strategy to decrease cost and duration and hospitalization. *Cathet Cardiovasc Diagn* 1992; 25:290–292.
25. Litvack F, Margolis J, Cummins F, Bresnahan J, Goldenberg T, Rothbaum D, King S, Holmes D, Block P, Douglas J, Forrester J for the ELCA Investigators: Excimer Laser Coronary (ELCA) Registry: report of the first consecutive 2080 patients. *J Am Coll Cardiol* 1992; 19:276A.
26. Popma JJ, Topol EJ, Hinohara T, Pinkerton CA, Baim DS, King SB III, Holmes DR Jr, Whitlow PL, Kereiakes DJ, Hartzler GO, Kent KM, Ellis SG, Simpson JB: Abrupt vessel closure after directional coronary atherectomy. *J Am Coll Cardiol* 1992; 19:1372–1379.
27. Buchbinder M, Leon M, Warth D, Marco J, Dorros G, Zacca N, Erbel R: Multicenter registry of percutaneous coronary rotational ablation using the Rotablator. *J Am Coll Cardiol* 1992: 19:333A.
28. Sketch MH Jr, O'Neill WW, Galichia JP, Feldman RC, Walker CM, Sawchak SR, Meany TB, Wall TC, O'Connor CM, Tcheng JE, Phillips HR, Stack RS: Restenosis following coronary transluminal extraction-endarterectomy: the final analysis of a multicenter registry. *J Am Coll Cardiol* 1992; 19–277A.
29. Black AJR, Anderson V, Roubin GS, Powelson SW, Douglas JS, King SB: Repeat coronary angioplasty: correlates of a second restenosis. *J Am Coll Cardiol* 1988; 11:714–718.
30. Teirstein PS, Hoover CA, Ligon RW, Georgi LV, Rutherford BD, McConahay DR, Johnson WL, Hartzler GO: Repeat coronary angioplasty: efficacy of a third angioplasty for a second restenosis. *J Am Coll Cardiol* 1989; 13:291–296.
31. Savage M, Fischman D, Leon M, Ellis S, Schatz R, Goldberg S: Restenosis risk of single Plamaz-Schatz stents in native coronaries: report from the Core Angiographic Laboratory. *J Am Coll Cardiol* 1992; 19:277A.

CHAPTER 12

Interfacial Relationships and Future Design Considerations

Julio C. Palmaz

A deeper understanding of the mechanisms of interaction of intravascular metallic stent and the host environment may help to improve the performance of these devices in clinical practice. Immediately after exposure of a metallic surface with circulating blood, a series of events modify such surface in preparation for tissue colonization. These events occur in rapid succession initially, and then much more slowly to finally reach a seemingly quiescent state years after stent placement. Much of the biological host response to intravascular stenting depends on the chemical composition of the device, its surface characteristics, and its mechanical properties. The thrombotic phenomena occurring after stent placement take center-stage attention and require knowledge of the intricacies of thrombogenicity and its prevention and treatment. Since the ultimate goal of stenting is to achieve total endothelialization of the surface to protect against slow-flow thrombosis, meticulous preservation of endothelium during implantation results in obvious benefit. This chapter does not provide an exhaustive examination of these issues but attempts an introduction to the most important ones.

Metallic Composition and Surface Characteristics

A number of intravascular devices that have been in widespread use for years provide useful experience about biocompatibility of certain alloys and pure metals. Although the devices in Table 1 have different basic functions including vessel occlusion, filtration, and stenting, a large clinical experience attests to the biocompatible properties of their material compositions. The most common alloys used for intravascular devices are the medical-grade stainless

From: Herrmann HC, Hirshfeld JW, eds. *Clinical Use of the Palmaz-Schatz Intracoronary Stent.* Futura Publishing Company, Inc., Mount Kisco, NY, © 1993.

Table 1.
Metallic Composition of Intravascular Devices

Z stent	304 stainless steel
Palmaz stent	316L stainless steel
Medinvent stent	Mediloy (?)
Strecker stent	Tantalum
Nitinol stent	Nitinol
Greenfield filter	316L stainless steel, B3Ti
Birdsnest filter	304 stainless steel
Gunter filter	304 stainless steel
Gianturco coils	304 stainless steel

From: Teitelbaum GP et al., *Radiology* 1988; 166:657.

Table 2.
Atomic Composition of Stainless-Steel Devices

	Composition (%)							
Stainless Steel	*C*	*Mn*	*P*	*S*	*Si*	*Cr*	*Ni*	*Mo*
304	0.08	2	0.045	0.03	1	18	10	—
316L	0.03	2	0.045	0.03	1	18	14	2.5

steels, also designated as 300 series. The 304 and 316L stainless steels are eight- and nine-element alloys, respectively of which, in addition to iron, chromium accounts for a sizable part of their bulk composition. Other components such as molybdenum in 316L account for only a small percentage (Table 2), but have important roles to stabilize the crystallographic phases, and to determine physical characteristics. The finish process of a device influences its biocompatiblity because it may determine the chemical characteristics of the surface. Electropolishing, a very common finish process for 300 stainless steels, removes most of the elements from the metal surface, leaving a high concentration of chromium, which accounts for the shiny, mirrorlike finish of the device. After exposure to air and a sterilization process, chromium reacts with oxygen to create a layer of oxide a few Angstrom's thick that stabilizes the surface and prevents further oxidation. Similar phenomena occur with tantalum, titanium, and other metals; therefore, in all intravascular devices a layer of metal oxide will provide the ultimate interfacial relationship with the host after implantation.

Initial Events After Stent Implantation

Most of the reactivity of metals, when placed in contact with circulating blood, depends on physical characteristics of the metal surface.[1] The most important one, because it can be altered by the manufacturing process, is surface texture. The rougher the surface the higher the thrombogenicity, so the thrombogenic properties of a device can be improved by attaining the highest degree of surface smoothness possible. Surface electrical charge or rest potential is apparently important since the metals and alloys used for most intravascular devices are electropositive in electrolytic solutions, while all biological intravascular phases are negatively charged. However, this positive electrical potential may be responsible for initial attraction of blood proteins which cover the surface to a thickness of 50 Angstroms of fibrinogen in a few seconds. This α-helical, random-tangle layer increases in thickness with time, and substitutes the highly thrombogenic metal surface by a less thrombogenic protein layer.[2] This event, known as passivation, may be viewed as a beneficial process. Another surface property which imparts metal reactivity with blood is free surface energy. It is related to unsatisfied intermolecular bonds at a cut surface which define the behavior of liquids when in contact with this surface. This interaction determines whether a fluid droplet spreads or not over a solid surface as a function of its wettability. A measure of this property is the critical surface tension. For a solid surface to be relatively thromboresistant the critical surface tension must be between 20 to 40 dynes per cm. Most clean metals have higher critical surface tensions and are therefore thrombogenic when evaluated for this particular property. Fortunately, the fibrinogen layer, which rapidly passivates the metal surface, has a critical surface tension within the thromboresistant range, providing a relative protection in this respect.

Endothelialization of the Stented Surface

After dilatation and stenting of a stenotic lesion it is possible that some endothelial cells remain on the luminal surface of the vessel wall between the stent struts. These remaining patches of endothelium and the ostia of side branches arising from the stented segment may provide sites for multicentric spread and complete coverage of the stent. Experimental evidence supports this contention and demonstrates that endothelial cells proliferate eccentrically to bridge over fibrin-covered struts[3] (Fig. 1). It is logical to assume that stenting of a previously occluded segment or a stenotic lesion that has been treated by atherectomy, laser or any other tissue-removal therapy leaves a surface totally devoid of endothelium. Endothelialization must proceed in this case from the ends of the stented segment and must be consequently a slower process (Fig. 2). Two mechanical characteristics of the stent that have an important role in stent endothelialization are resistance to hoop or circumferential stress and total metal-to-free surface ratio of the expanded stent. The first one affects the profile of the stented surface since a "strong" stent will exert enough radial pressure to cause embedment of the struts and decrease metal exposure. A small metal-to-free surface ratio is desirable, provided that the stented lumen remains cylindrical. Surface irregularities from a stent with large spaces between struts will induce deposition of thrombus, eventually reducing the lumi-

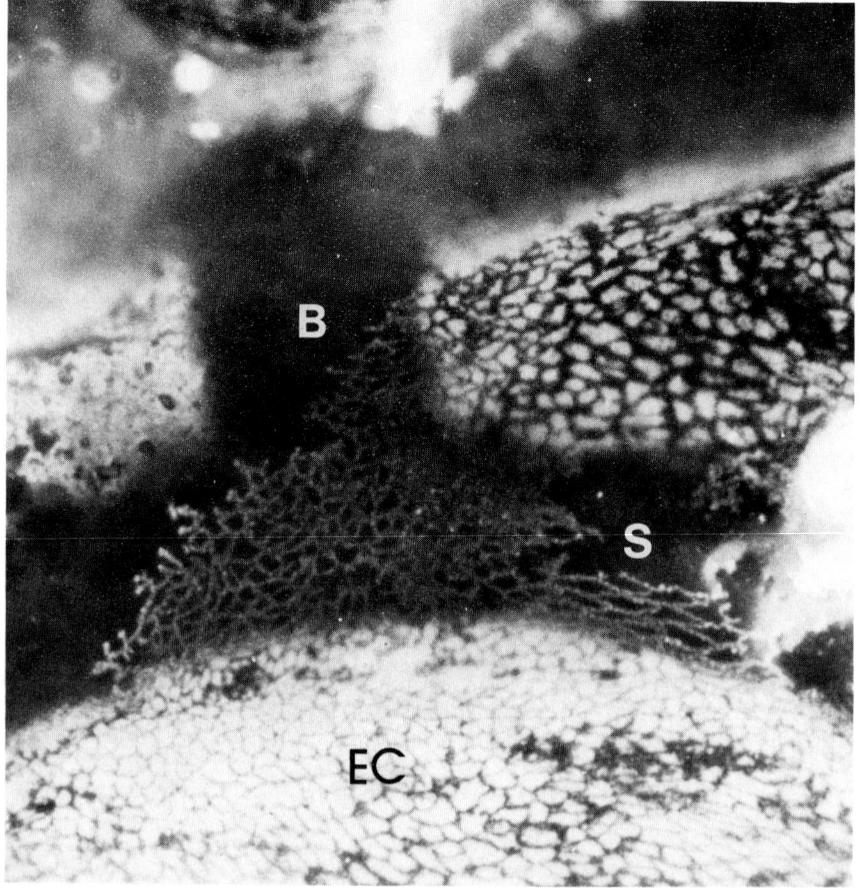

Figure 1: *Endothelial cells growing over intersection of strut and bridge of stent, 3 days after placement in rabbit aorta. (S = strut; B = bridge; EC = endothelial cells; Transillumination, silver nitrate stain x 125). Reproduced with permission from, AJR 1988; 150:1266).*

nal area. Since an increase in hoop strength involves an increase in metal bulk causing an increase of metal surface, the relationship between hoop strength and metal surface must be a compromise, and it can be described as "stenting ability."

Metal-Cell Interaction

In days to weeks, the fibrin layer covering the stent struts is progressively replaced by fibromuscular tissue. Replacement occurs first around struts and coincides with development of new vessels, suggesting that the neointimal cells arrive from blood-borne precursors. Eventually all thrombotic material

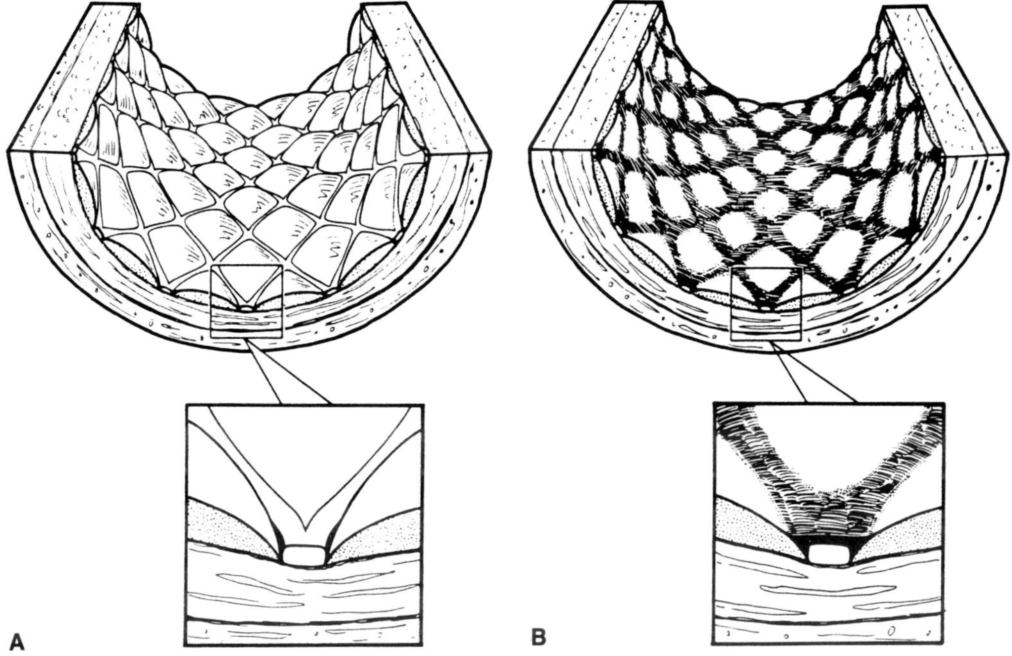

Figure 2: (A) Correct placement of an intravascular stent is obtained by embedding the metal members in the arterial wall. Tissue mounds protrude between the struts. **(B)** Thrombus rapidly fills the depressions, leaving portions of the arterial wall exposed. The protrusions of the wall may contain endothelial cells that survived instrumentation.

is replaced by fibromuscular cells and intercellular matrix. In experimental situations, this tissue reaches maximum thickness at 8 weeks and is then progressively replaced by collagen[4] (see Chapter 1). Stent neointima examined 6 years after stenting is predominantly composed of collagen with scattered fibrocytes. It is possible that this scarring process causes thinning of the neointima and enlargement of the lumen. This was seen in experimental observations but has not been proven in clinical practice. Cells in direct contact with the metal surface develop a strong physical attachment to it. Chemical bonds developing between the glycoproteins of the glycocalyx and the oxide layer of the metal account for such attachment. It is possible that the metal surface induces cell proliferation by leaching out ions that may act as cofactors in enzymatic processes involved in cell replication and synthesis.[5] Whether this is the only factor governing the cycle of proliferation followed by atrophy is not known.

Flexibility Versus Rigidity: Radial Compliance

Radial compliance has long been considered an important factor for preservation of patency in surgical bypass material. Compliance mismatch between

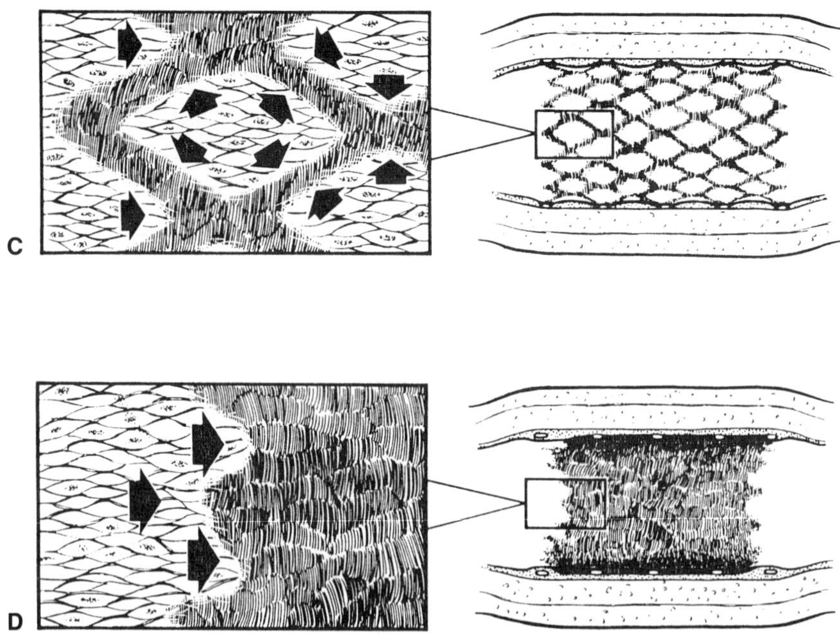

Figures 2C,D: (C) Endothelial regeneration proceeds in a multicentric fashion. Since the endothelial gaps are limited to the stent struts covered by thrombus, confluence may occur more rapidly. **(D)** A stent not embedded protrudes into the lumen causing increased thrombus deposition. The entire stented surface is covered with continuous thrombus. Endothelialization must proceed from the ends of this surface and is, therefore, a slower process.

host vessel and prosthetic conduit has been blamed for anastamotic intimal hyperplasia and graft failure.[6] This has led to industrial efforts to produce bypass material with radial compliance similar to that of arteries. This seems futile since prosthetic material becomes rigid after the fibroblastic healing process reduces its compliance.

One of the most controverted issues in intravascular stenting is the relevance of longitudinal flexibility in the maintenance of long-term patency. There is little argument that longitudinal flexibility is desirable for stent placement as it enables negotiating around complex delivery catheter shapes and curved vessels. However, longitudinal stent motion may affect long-term stent patency by negatively influencing the stability of the neointima and the endothelial cover. The endothelium growing on the fibrinous layer is likely to be quite susceptible to slough if the substrate where it is based is subject to the dimensional changes imposed by flexion and extension. This is supported by previous experience demonstrating improved patency of saphenous coronary bypass grafts if they were rendered rigid by the placement of an external, constrictive mesh. The endothelium of meshed grafts appeared more mature and exhibited less cellular attachment and the underlying intima was thinner.[7]

Barth[8] recently compared the intimal thickness of rigid and flexible stents placed in common femoral arteries of dogs where substantial longitudinal motion occurred. The mean intimal area of the rigid stents was significantly smaller than that of flexible stents. Motion may also have a direct effect on the neointimal cells that may affect the neointimal thickness. Leung et al[9] demonstrated that myofibroblasts exposed to cyclic stretching increased their synthetic activity severalfold as compared to stationary cells.

The Stent of the Future

Although the mainstay of intravascular stenting is the permanently implanted metal stent, other avenues are being explored that depart from this concept. Stents made of polylactic and polyglycolic acid and other absorbable materials have been proposed to combine the tissue-remodeling effects of stenting and the avoidance of a permanent prosthetic implant.[10] These materials, widely used in resorbable surgical sutures and staples, have markedly lower mechanical strength than "surgical" metals and alloys. This will require a substantial increase in the bulk of stents made of such resorbable materials to approximate the mechanical performance of metal stents. Also, it is possible that by the time the resorbable stent has disappeared from the treated site, the atrophic changes that invariably occur after the musculoelastic elements of the arterial wall are put to rest, may lead to aneurysmal dilatation. The increased bulk limitation may be relevant in small vessels while the risk of aneurysmal formation and rupture would be of concern in large vessels.

Temporary stenting is another way to avoid a permanent implant. The goal of temporary stenting is to relieve acute vessel occlusion caused by instrumentation by placing a device that would exert temporary stenting action while allowing flow to proceed through the lumen. The Gaspard[11] stent, which remains attached to the catheter after deployment, consists of a wire device resembling a stone-retrieval basket. The removable stent from the University of Pennsylvania[12] detaches from the delivery catheter after deployment, but can be retrieved and extracted. The relocatable stent from Tokorasawa, Japan[13] can be withdrawn into the delivery catheter by hooking an encircling string for repositioning of the stent. Although the principle of temporary stenting is attractive, the inherent complexity of these devices and the added trauma involved in the retrieval process may compound their thrombogenicity, offsetting their advantage.

Coating of the metal surface to antagonize its thrombogenic properties has received widespread attention, and significant efforts have been devoted to achieve this goal. In general, stent coatings may be classified into prosthetic and biological coating. Prosthetic coatings may be subdivided into passive and active. Passive coatings are composed of materials such as pyrolytic carbon and urethanes with decreased thrombogenicity because of their favorable surface characteristics as compared to metals. Active coatings include several new materials with the ability to incorporate drugs such as low-molecular weight heparin for slow release or local action. Biological coatings are represented by endothelial-cell seeding over the stent surface prior to deployment. Dicheck et al[14] reported successful seeding of endothelium over stents, with a significant proportion of cells remaining attached to the surface after stent placement. Furthermore, these endothelial cells were genetically engineered by recombinant-DNA techniques to produce t-PA. This preliminary study was quite encouraging by identifying a number of future possibilities for intravascular stenting.

Although antithrombogenic coatings have already been tried in clinical practice, they have not shown a particular advantage. "Biogold"-coated Wallstents have not proved less thrombogenic than their noncoated counterparts.[15] Even if a coating that effectively decreases the thrombogenicity of metallic stents can be developed, questions remain about its effects on endothelialization and long-term patency. One may speculate that by antagonizing fibrin deposition over the stent struts the endothelial cell coverage may be slowed or impeded. Also, the composite nature of coated stents would pose additional engineering challenges in regard to long-term endurance and integrity. Of course, these considerations will not deter research which ultimately will answer these questions.

Metal stents have been proven safe and efficacious for large vessels such as the iliac arteries, and performance seems to improve continuously for smaller vessels as patient selection, anticoagulation regimens, and delivery systems improve. New research about stents seems to be focusing on improving current stent design and delivery systems as growing clinical experience defines the role of these devices.

REFERENCES

1. DePalma VA, Baier RE, Ford JW, Gott VL, and Furuse A: Investigation of three-surface properties of several metals and their relationship to blood compatibility. *J Biomed Mater Res* 1972; 3:37–75.
2. Baier RE, Dutton RC: Initial events in interaction of blood with a foreign surface. *J Biomed Mater Res* 1969; 3:191–206.
3. Palmaz JC, Tio FO, Schatz RA, Alvarado R, Rees C, Garcia FS: Early endothelization of balloon-expandable stents: experimental observations. *J Intervent Radiol* 1988; 3:119–124.
4. Schatz RA, Palmaz JC, Tio FO, Garcia FJ, Reuter SR: Balloon-expandable intracoronary stents in the adult dog. *Circulation* 1987; 76:450–457.
5. Gristina AG: Biomaterial centered infection: microbiol adhesion versus tissue integration. *Science* 1987; 237:1588–1595.
6. Abbott WM, Megerman J, Hasson JE, C'Italien G, Warnook DF: Effect of compliance mismatch on vascular graft patency. *J Vasc Surg* 1987:376–382.
7. Barra JA, Volant A, Leroy JP, Braesco J, Airiav J, Boschet J, Blanc JJ, Denther P: Constrictive perivenous mesh prosthesis for preservation of vein integrity. *J Thorac Cardiovasc Surg* 1986; 92:330–336.
8. Barth K: The effect of compliance mismatch on vascular stents. SCVIR 17th Annual Meeting, Washington, D.C., April 4–9, 1992.

9. Leung DYM, Glagon S, Mathews MD: Cyclic stretching stimulates synthesis of matrix components by arterial smooth muscle cells in vitro. *Science* 1976; 191: 475–477.
10. Slepian MJ, Schindler A: Polymeric endoluminal paring/sealing: a biodegradable alternative to intracoronary stenting. *Circulation* 1988; 78(suppl 2):II-409.
11. Gaspard PE, Didier BP, Delsanti GL: The temporary stent catheter: a nonoperative treatment for acute occlusion during coronary angioplasty. *J Am Coll Cardiol* 1990: 1S:118A.
12. Schlansky-Goldberg RD, LeVeen RF, Hillstead RA, Cope C: Temporary vascular stenting. *Radiology* 1990: 177(P):299. Abstract.
13. Irie T, Furui S, Yamauchi T, Makita K, Sawada S, Takenaka E: Relocatable Gianturco expandable metallic stents. *Radiology* 1991; 178:575–578.
14. Dichek DA, Neville RF, Zwiebel JA, Freeman SM, Leon MB, Anderson WF: Seeding of intravascular stents with genetically engineered endothelial cells. *Circulation* 1989; 80:1347–1353.
15. Wilms GE, Peene PT, Baert AL, Nevelsteen AA, Soy RM, Veahaeghe RH, Vermylen JG, Fagard RH: Renal artery stent placement with use of the Wallstent endoprosthesis. *Radiology* 1991; 179:457–462.

Index